ACID REFLUX

DIET

FOR BEGINNERS

*An Easy Cookbook With Low Acidic Recipes
Including Vegan, Gluten, GERD & LPR.*

By

DANIELLE T. CLOVER

Particular creators claim all copyrights not held by the distributor.

The data in this is offered for educational purposes exclusively and is all-inclusive as so. The introduction of the data is without a contract or any assurance confirmation.

The trademarks that are utilized are with no assent, and the distribution of the trademark is without consent or support by the trademark proprietor. All trademarks and brands inside this book are for explaining purposes just and are possessed by the proprietors, not partnered with this record.

TABLE OF CONTENTS

INTRODUCTION..5

WHAT ACID REFLUX CAUSES (GERD)?..........................8

WHAT CAUSES GERD?...9

SPECIFIC FOODS AND DR.INKS...................................11

WEIGHT PROBLEMS..16

ACID REFLUX SYMPTOMS (GERD).............................52

TREATMENT OPTIONS FOR ACID REFLUX.................68

WHAT DOES ACID REFLUX (GERD) FEEL LIKE?........69

UX (GERD) DIET...70

FOOD TO THE ACID REFLUX DIET............................108

LESS THAN 30 DAY TREATMENT AND RECIPES FOR ACID REFLUX..116

27 DAYS GASTRIC REFLUX DIET RECIPES...............122

NATURAL CURES FOR ACID REFLUX: HEALTHY ACID REFLUX TREATMENT..270

HOME REMEDIES TREAT AND SOOTH ACID REFLUX..279

CONCLUSION...285

DISCLAIMER..286

INTRODUCTION

A hot burning in the breast, a bitter preference in the throat, a fizzy bloating in the tummy-- heartburn is no picnic. What you consume, nonetheless, can have an influence. The best, as well as worst foods for indigestion, might mean the distinction in between wonderful relief and also sour suffering.

If you obtain heartburn, you know exactly how uncomfortable the feeling can be. In spite of attempting to remove the right foods, you still might be experiencing heartburn, so it's handy to know what foods can really deal with heartburn. What you consume is very important when it pertains to stopping gastrointestinal problems, as well as specific foods, can function marvels to alleviate discomfort and avoid future problems.

60% of the adult populace will certainly experience some kind of gastro oesophagus reflux disease each year, as well as 20 to 30% will certainly have weekly signs, according to Healthline. What precisely causes these symptoms?

Acid reflux occurs when tummy acid leaks up, the wrong direction, from the stomach right into the oesophagus. Signs of indigestion variety from heartburn to problem ingesting - or there can be no signs and symptoms in all. It can be unpleasant, bothersome, and uneasy to the victim.

Trickey consistently sees clients in her centre dealing with heartburn, and also has actually located that the most significant contributor to reflux is actually just how people consume. 'Most people consume rapidly, do not chew their food correctly, and have a tendency to eat while persistently doing various other things, so they are not relaxed when they consume,' claims Trickey. 'Yet food digestion works best when the body is relaxed.'

' Overeating is additionally a huge issue when it comes to reflux,' she adds. 'Especially when eating in restaurants as portion dimensions are normally way also huge. Individuals fail to remember that their tummy is just the size of their clenched fist. Many of us try to fit way extra food than that in there!'

What Is Gastrooesophagus Reflux Disease (GERD)?

Gastrooesophagus reflux disease (GERD) is a problem in which the oesophagus ends up being aggravated or swollen due to acid backing up from the tummy. The oesophagus or food pipeline is television extending from the throat to the tummy. It travels down the oesophagus when food is ingested.

The belly produces Dr. chloric acid after a meal to help in the food digestion of food.

The inner cellular lining of the stomach withstands corrosion by this acid. The cells lining the tummy secrete large quantities of safety mucous.

The cellular lining of the oesophagus does not share these immune attributes, as well as stomach acid, which can harm it.

The oesophagus exists just behind the heart, so the term "heartburn" was coined to describe the feeling of acid shedding the oesophagus near where the heart is located.

Usually, a ring of muscular tissue at the bottom of the oesophagus, called the reduced oesophagus sphincter, stops reflux (or supporting) of acid.

This sphincter relaxes throughout swallowing to permit food to pass. It then tightens up to prevent flow in the opposite direction.

With GERD, nonetheless, the sphincter kicks back between swallows, enabling belly materials (gastric reflux) and corrosive acid to well up and damage the lining of the oesophagus.

GERD impacts 20% of the US populace. Not only grownups are affected; even babies, as well as chilDr.en, can have GERD.

WHAT ACID REFLUX CAUSES (GERD)?

After ingested food travels down the oesophagus, it promotes cells in the tummy to produce acid and also pepsin (an enzyme), which helps digestion. A band of muscle at the reduced component of the oesophagus, called the reduced oesophagus sphincter (LES), functions as an obstacle to prevent the back-flow (reflux) of stomach materials right into the oesophagus. The LES normally kicks back to enable ingested food to enter the tummy.

Reflux happens when that obstacle is unwinded at improper times, is weak, or is or else jeopardized. In addition, factors such as delayed stomach dislocation of the tummy, large moving Hiatal hernia, or excessive acid in the stomach can make indigestion much easier.

WHAT CAUSES GERD?

There is no well-known solitary reason for gastro oesophagus reflux illness (GERD). It occurs when the oesophagal defences are bewildered by gastric materials that reflux into the oesophagus.

Gastrooesophagus reflux takes place when the LES obstacle is somehow endangered. Periodic reflux occurs typically, as well as without effect besides irregular heartburn, in people who do not have GERD. In individuals with GERD, reflux creates frequent symptoms or problems in the oesophagal cells.

Some, yet not all, people with Hiatal rupture have GERD and also vice versa. The LES can threaten the ability to avoid acid reflux if the diaphragm is not intact.

Also, when the LES, as well as the diaphragm, are undamaged and also operating usually, reflux can still happen. The LES might unwind after having big meals resulting in distension of the upper part of the stomach. When that takes place, there is not nearly enough stress at the LES to avoid reflux. In some patients, the LES is also weak or can not install enough pressure to prevent reflux throughout durations of enhanced pressure within the abdomen.

The level of injury to the oesophagus-- and the level of severity of GERD-- depends on the frequency of reflux, the amount of time the refluxed material remains in the oesophagus, as well as the quantity of acid in the oesophagus.

There are lots of aspects that affect the symptoms of GERD.

If the reflux becomes frequent and extreme sufficient, you may have gastro oesophagus reflux conditions (GERD). While this needs to be dealt with to stay clear of issues (including a higher risk of oesophagal cancer), you can typically deal with or perhaps avoid occasional acid reflux on your own with a way of living modifications like consuming smaller dishes as well as shedding excess weight. Here are several of the much more regular sources of the problem.

SPECIFIC FOODS AND DR.INKS

Many individuals complain that they obtain reflux after consuming certain foods. Common offenders include things high in fat, chocolate, zesty foods, citrusy, or acidic foods like oranges as well as tomatoes, mint, garlic, as well as onions, along with soft Dr.inks.

These foods might be more difficult to digest, generating extra tummy acid that can wind up in the oesophagus. The lower oesophagus sphincter (LES) can also be released from fatty foods, which normally act as a "lid." Elena Ivanina, D.O. MPH, the gastroenterologist at Lenox Hill in New York, explains, "The LES prevents acid backflow from tube to oesophagal." Sometimes, however, LES does not perform its work beside it.

Medical professionals typically guidance lifestyle modifications-- including avoiding these triggering foods-- to battle reflux signs prior to attempting Dr.ugs. Dr. Schiller, also the program coordinator of the Gastroenterology Fellowship at Baylor College of Medicine in Dallas, says: "This is something people can do without wasting large sums on medicine.

Foods That Cause Acid Reflux

There are certain foods that are nearly globally bothersome when it comes to acid reflux. The best strategy is to prevent them, yet they commonly comprise over half of many individuals' diets.

Chocolate

Chocolate problems seem to be causing more reflux than any other kind of food. It is a tri-strong whom: Delicious chocolate contains theobromine, which triggers reflux, and other stimulants.

Delicious fatty chocolate and fat causes reflux

For cacao, too, chocolate is strong, and cacao induces reflux.

Dark chocolate is a theory not so poor as high-fat milk chocolate, but let's admit it — all delicious recalcitrant chocolate.

Soft Dr.ink

soda-caffeine

Soda and also other carbonated beverages are a few of the primary causes of indigestion. The bubbles of carbonation expand inside the belly, and the boosted pressure adds to reflux. Sodas with high levels of caffeine, as well as those that are acidic (mostly all), are also worse.

Coke, Tab, and Diet Pepsi have been among the most acidic beverages tested. Any carbonated beverages may be a problem, so the authors suggest to refrain completely from acid reflux.

Fried food

The most well-known cause of reflux is fried food. It is also the food often associated with a cardiac burn, which is oesophagus pain in the upper body.

Because of their high ingredients, deep-fried (or even not so deep-fried) food comes on the "negational checklist."

Alcohol

Beer, liquor, and also red wine is believed to add to reflux. Lots of alcoholic beverages are not very acidic. Nonetheless, alcohol is believed to relax the shutoff at the end of the oesophagus (where it joins the tummy), leading to reflux.

Take care, if possible; otherwise, only one glass of wine a day or a cocktail and also avoid acid mixers like orange or soda completely .

High-fat milk items

All high-fat foods trigger reflux. There is no factor in thinking that high-fat butter or cheese is better than an additional hereof. If you have reflux and a major cheese habit, something needs to offer.

Utilize a percentage of these foods as flavouring, however, not as cornerstones. Slim is much better than no fat.

High-fat meats

Indigestion is triggered by high-fat cuts of meat-- beef, pork, lamb-- which remain longer in the tummy as well as increase the possibility of indigestion.

Try reducing to a lean cut of meat and also consume it only when a week.

High levels of caffeine

One cup of coffee or coffee a day is fine, yet people that consume coffee all day are dating reflux-- if they do not have it already.

Try switching to chamomile, which is the most effective organic tea, or you can have one mug of environment-friendly tea a day if it is gently made.

WEIGHT PROBLEMS

Weight problems are one of the primary chauffeurs behind both acid reflux as well as GERD. It might also enhance the threat of GERD complications like Barrett's oesophagus, a problem entailing precancerous adjustments in oesophagal cells.

It's not simply added fat that appears to elevate the danger. It's "main obesity," which indicates more fat around your centre, states Dr. Ivanina.

Professionals believe extra stomach fat adds stress to the stomach, requiring acid up into the oesophagus. Hormonal agents might likewise play a role. People that are overweight have more flowing estrogen, which has been related to GERD signs and symptoms. Postmenopausal females utilizing hormone treatment also have a boosted risk of reflux.

Research studies have actually shown that reducing weight either with diet plan and exercise or bariatric surgical treatment can ease signs of reflux.

Weight management and also acid reflux

Being overweight is connected to several health and wellness issues. These include depression, fatigue, and also a raised risk of chronic diseases, such as heart disease. Another illness related to excess weight is indigestion or heartburn. Recognizing the link between excess pounds and also acid reflux can assist you to take procedures to maintain your weight. This can provide alleviation for your heartburn.

It is usual to understand that certain foods can cause gastro oesophagus reflux (GERD)—a condition identified by constant heartburn episodes.

However, physicians, as well as scientists, have actually shown in a variety of various researches that excess body weight-- also being simply slightly overweight-- can also activate the start of GERD as well as influence its extent.

Likewise, there's evidence that losing excess body weight can boost or even settle signs of GERD.

It's uncertain exactly why additional body weight has a result on GERD, yet one likely explanation is that the added weight puts pressure on your abdomen. This boosts the risk that your reduced oesophagus sphincter (LES)-- the ring of muscle mass in between your oesophagus as well as stomach-- will loosen up when it shouldn't.

Another feasible explanation is that people with a greater body weight may eat extra fat, which is a well-known GERD trigger.

It might be rewarding to talk to your medical professional about just how losing weight could boost your signs if you have GERD and you're overweight or overweight.

In heartburn, also called GERD (gastro oesophagus reflux disease), tummy acid recedes right into the oesophagus, the tube leading from the throat to the stomach.

Obesity raises the danger of GERD,and also two other problems-- abrasive esophagitis as well as cancer of the oesophagus-- create Howard Hampel, MD, as well as colleagues.

The Hampel team works at the Michael E. DeBakey Veteran Affairs Medical Center in Houston Baylor College of Medicine. The Internal Medicine Annals are record-breaking.

GERD-Obesity Link

The scientists analyzed 9types of research done from 1966 to 2004. 6 research studies revealed a notable link between excessive weight and also GERD.

" The association in between BMI as well as GERD difficulties was markedly regular," write the scientists. None of the research studies revealed any GERD gain from weight problems, and the research studies that didn't strongly link weight problems and also GERD slanted because instructions, they write.Check Your Heartburn SymptomsCheck Your Heartburn Symptoms.

In 8 of the nine types of research, as BMI (body mass index-- a procedure of body fat) rose, so did GERD signs, compose the scientists, who set quality criteria for the studies they reviewed.

Tiny Weight Gain Linked to GERD

A vital research study on GERD and body weight was released in The New England Journal of Medicine (NEJM).

In this research, researchers looked for to figure out whether reasonably little modifications in body weight-- even within the bounds of typical weight-- can impact the seriousness of indigestion and also related signs in women.

A clear link between BMI and GERD signs and symptoms was found in this study.The scientists discovered that ladies who were obese- defined by a body mass index of 25 to 30-- were greater than twice as likely to establish heartburn as those of normal weight.

Women who were obese-- with a BMI higher than 30-- had virtually three-way the threat of GERD signs, like heartburn, acid regurgitation, breast pain, and also trouble ingesting.

Perhaps most surprising, though, was that tiny differences in body weight in ladies of typical weight-- with a BMI of 21 to 25-- likewise influenced the probability of creating GERD.

Also, in females that began with typical body weight, an increase in BMI of greater than 3.5 was associated with almost three-way the risk of experiencing constant GERD symptoms.

Out of 10,545 females in the study, 22% reported at least once weekly GERD-signs and symptoms. 55 per cent have had both heartburn and acid regurgitation amongst those with symptoms.

The researchers in this research study emphasized that people with GERD whose body weight is optimal shouldn't try to slim down. If you've gotten weight as well as noticed an increase in your symptoms, you may be able to reverse this scenario by shedding the weight once again.

Weight-loss Programs for GERD

There's strong proof that if you're obese, participating in an organized fat burning program can assist relieve signs of GERD.

In a research released in March 2013 in the journal Obesity, 332 overweight adults participated in a program that consisted of nutritional modifications, raised exercise, as well as behaviour strategies. (2) After 6 months, 97 per cent had reduced weight, with a typical loss of 13 kgs (29 extra pounds).

The incidence of GERD in the group decreased from 37% to 15% during the same period, with 81% of people experiencing decreases in their GERD symptoms. Greater weight loss was linked to a greater decline of GERD symbols, even though females lost only 5 to 10percent of their cardiovascular weight during the study.

Researchers examined a weight management program called The Reflux Improvement as well as Monitoring program (TRIM) which gave participants "personalised, multidisciplinary" health education and learning as well as monitoring, over a period of six months, in one more research study, published in October 2017 in The American Journal of gastroenterology.

Because of this, participants-- a team of 52 obese individuals-- seasoned significantly greater weight management 3, 6, and 12 months after beginning the program as compared with a similar team that really did not register in the program.

Amongst TRIM participants, scores showing GERD sign seriousness Dr.opped considerably after three months, as well as remained significantly down after 6 months. At the exact same time, ratings showing GERD-related lifestyle additionally boosted, however not to a statistically considerable degree-- indicating that this renovation can have been because of chance.

This tiny research study revealed that a multidisciplinary weight loss program intended at individuals with GERD could result in weight loss, improved signs and symptoms, as well as overall fulfilment with the program.

Hiatal hernia

A Hiatal hernia is when the leading part of your stomach protrudes up right into your dental breast caries, protecting against the LES from closing appropriately.

Lots of people with Hiatal hernias have no signs in all. In various other situations, the rupture can be brought on by GERD, and also in still others, GERD is a symptom of the hernia.

Hiatal hernias are much more usual after the age of 50 and also in people that are overweight. They often also happen after coughing, throwing up, or a physical injury.

Slimming down along with a healthy and balanced diet plan can aid in regulating reflux signs due to a Hiatal rupture. Some individuals with reflux because of Hiatal hernias might take advantage of over the counter or prescription heartburn medications. In severe instances, surgery may be required to press the tummy to pull back as well as reinforce the barrier between the oesophagus and also the belly.

Comprehending the Link Between Hiatal Hernia and also GERD

Explaining the relationship between Hiatal hernias as well as gastro oesophagus reflux condition (GERD), doctors claim, resembles describing the "chicken or the egg" situation.

"People could experience a Hiatal hernia without GERD. Whether the Hiatal rupture has created GERD is not uncertain in both."According to guide, Hiatal Hernia Surgery, published in August 2017, suggests that the partnership between these problems is reasonably intertwined and also has clinical value.

Individuals with a Hiatal hernia might be extra likely to have GERD. There is also a close connection between Hiatal hernia size as well as the occurrence of GERD.

Leslie Memsic, MD, a surgical oncologist that specializes in breast cancer cells as well as hernia therapy at the Bedford Breast Center in Beverly Hills, claims some research studies suggest that chronic acid reflux actually brings about the weakening of the sphincter and also the advancement of a Hiatal hernia. "But, extra generally, a big Hiatal rupture is believed to contribute to GERD," Dr Memsic claims.

Is the GERD or the Hiatal Hernia?

A Hiatal hernia can happen from lasting GERD or GERD can be a sign of a Hiatal rupture, according to the Cleveland Clinic. When GERD progresses, it can trigger the reduced oesophagus sphincter to lose its function, which may cause a Hiatal rupture, according to RefluxMD.

The diaphragm (rest) void triggers a Hiatal hernia when food and liquids migrate from the oesophagus straight into the abdomen.This facilitates indigestion and also can trigger the tummy to slide upwards into the upper body, says Dr. Castro. This problem in extreme situations can cause much more severe problems such as blockage or strangulation of the belly, says Memsic.

Deteriorated muscles in the diaphragm can permit the stomach to relocate freely into the respite, or inherited architectural irregularities in the diaphragm can cause a congenital Hiatal rupture, which provides at birth. Maternity, as well as obesity, are likewise risk elements for Hiatal hernia, according to the Mayo Clinic.

GERD is very typical and typically provides as heartburn, a condition that affects more than 40 per cent of Americans. GERD occurs when "belly materials reflux back into the oesophagus, triggering issues such as heartburn, regurgitation, difficulty swallowing. And even breast discomfort is the presence of stomach materials in the oesophagus,"

Tiny Hiatal ruptures do not commonly existing indicators or signs and symptoms, according to the Mayo Clinic, but those with an extra serious rupture may experience:

- Heartburn
- Regurgitation of food or liquids right into the mouth
- Backflow of stomach acid into the oesophagus (acid reflux).
- Trouble swallowing.
- Sickness in breast or belly.

- Shortness of breath.

In serious instances, a Hiatal hernia can cause blood loss, strangulation, and also the opening of the belly claims Castro.

A lot of people are truly rupturing Hiale without the GERD, and others also are GERD without the rupture of Hialeah. Most individuals have no signs and symptoms of Hialeah breakup. According to a report from the School of Medicine and Public Health of the University of Wisconsin, you suffer from a Hiale spin with constant and even more extreme signs and symptoms.

Eat a big meal and lie down afterwards

Eating a big meal at any moment can activate heartburn. However,it's particularly problematic if you do it right before you go to bed or choose to lounge on the couch.

Blame it on gravity. "Eating right prior to lying down results in reflux given that the stomach is complete while one is resting and it is much easier for the acid to support into the oesophagus," clarifies Dr. Ivanina. "Large meals additionally might conquer the oesophagus obstacle and lead to greater acid exposure."

Try eating numerous little meals startled throughout the day as opposed to less big meals. Don't lie down till 2 or three hours after you consume, and also, if you still have issues, try increasing the head of your bed a couple of inches to offset the impact of gravity.

" A lot of individuals get some remedy for sleeping on a slope or with a wedge under their body," claims Dr. Schiller.

Smoking cigarettes

Cigarette smoking can damage your digestive system just as it damages so many other parts of your body. Also used smoke, as well as a chewing cigarette, can contribute to reflux by loosening up the reduced oesophagus sphincter.

" Smoking as well as alcohol both contribute to reflux as they lower LES pressure, minimize acid clearance and also damage safety oesophagus features," states Dr Ivanina.

The study has shown that quitting smoking can boost reflux (as if you needed an additional reason to give up or not to start to begin with).

Smoking might additionally contribute to reflux by making you cough. "A lot of people that smoke coughing, as well as each time you cough, you're increasing stress in your belly and promoting reflux," claims Dr. Schiller.

Studies have closely linked cigarette smoking to GERD, and smokers suffering from continuous acid reflux commonly discover some remedy for their GERD once they stop.

The research study likewise has connected cigarette smoking to a few of the worst problems of GERD, consisting of Barrett's oesophagus as well as throat cancer cells.

Doctors claim that cigarette smoking contributes to GERD by:

The sphincter regulates the flow of food right into the belly, and also protects against acid from refluxing into the oesophagus. When nicotine causes the sphincter to unwind, there's a boosted threat of acid surging right into and damaging the oesophagus.

Decreasing salivation. Saliva contains an acid-neutralizing compound called bicarbonate, which aids in battle the results of heartburn as well as GERD. Primarily, when you ingest your saliva, it assists quell whatever acid damages are occurring due to reflux. Cigarette smokers generate much less saliva, and so have much less capability to counteract refluxed acid.

They have increased tummy acid secretion.Smoking prompts the stomach to produce even more acid, increasing the threat of gastric juices being refluxed into the oesophagus. Smoking cigarettes likewise seems to make tummy acid extra intense and destructive by advertising the transfer of bile salts from the intestines into the tummy.

I am disrupting the oesophagus muscular tissues. In kicking back smooth muscle mass, pure nicotine also can interfere with the muscular tissues that aid move food down the oesophagus. These muscles help free the oesophagus of harmful heartburn.

Damages cellular oesophagus. Smoking cigarettes are hazardous to layers of mucosa that prevent acid damage to the oesophagus.

Maternity

As lots of as fifty per cent of all pregnant females experience acid reflux. It can begin at any factor when you're anticipating, yet it's more common after 27 weeks.

" It's [typically] blamed on hormones," says Dr. Schiller. "The uterus grows and enhances stress on the stomach. Hormonal agents are greater, which tends to relax the sphincter."

You're more probable to have heartburn when you're expecting if you've had it before or if you've been pregnant previously.

Once anticipated, you are most effective in reducing the symptoms of acid reflux, paying close attention to your diet, and avoiding trigger foods. Talk to your physician before trying any kind of counter medication because not everybody is safe to take during pregnancy. After your baby is born, the reflux must subside.

Once you are expected to reduce acid reflux symptoms, pay close attention to your diet, and avoid trigger foods. Talk to your doctor before you try any counter Dr.ugs because not everyone is safe to take during pregnancy. The reflux must subside after your baby is born.

Why is it during pregnancy?

During pregnancy, the majority of women who have heartburn had never had problems. But, if you experienced heartburn, you would probably have symptoms before pregnancy. While the particular reasons are unclear, many experts believe that hormonal substances for pregnancy, in particular, progesterone, play a role. Hormones cause the leisure of the oesophagus sphincter. This is a tight circular band of muscular tissue on top of the belly. This permits partially digested food and also belly acids to backflow, or reflux, right into the oesophagus. In addition, progesterone additionally slows down the digestive process. This keeps food in the tummy longer. The pregnancy itself-- the upward stress of the growing womb-- likewise may play a role.

What makes it worse?

Overeating or consuming big dishes, in general, can additionally raise the danger for heartburn. Smoking makes heartburn even worse as well as is another factor to quit, particularly while expectant.

What makes it much better?

For most women, points that help in reducing acid production or prevent reflux are useful in preventing the discomfort of heartburn. Here are ideas that might assist:

Avoid classic zesty foods, as well as those with lots of fat or oil. Numerous individuals advise staying clear of citrus and also chocolate.

Eat numerous, small meals spread out throughout the day, much like "grazing," rather than 3 huge meals.

Attempt boosting the head of your bed by numerous inches, as well as wait a while after consuming before going to sleep or lying down.

Some females locate that it's far better to consume liquids between dishes, rather than with a dish. This can increase the number of components in the tummy.

They work by covering the lining of the oesophagus and also stomach and also neutralizing belly acid. Heartburn medicines called H2-blockers work by reducing the amount of acid made by your tummy.

Medications

Despite the fact that medications can amazingly eliminate much of what ails us as humans, they all have adverse effects. If you get regular heartburn, you might believe that food or beverage is responsible. The offender might actually be hiding in your bathroom: Certain discomfort relievers, as well as other usual medications, can create heartburn, the most typical signs and symptom of stomach reflux disease, additionally recognized as acid reflux.

Nearly everyone has experienced heartburn at one time or one more. Actually, virtually 40 per cent of Americans have heartburn signs a minimum of when a month.

Heartburn, as well as acid reflux,happen when acid or various other stomach contents back up into your oesophagus, the lengthy tube that brings food from your mouth to your belly. Often, heartburn triggers a sour taste in your mouth or a burning experience that may start under your breastbone before taking a trip as much as your throat.

In some instances, the lower oesophagus sphincter (LES), a ring of muscular tissue that assists keep food in the belly after you swallow, may also come to be weakened, enabling food and belly acid to take a trip back towards the mouth.

If you usually follow a healthy and balanced diet regimen however discover that you're experiencing heartburn, or if your heartburn signs and symptoms coincide with starting a Dr.ug, you might intend to look in your medication cupboard for possible perpetrators.

Heartburn Causes: Common Medications

The complying with typical medicines can cause or worsen heartburn:

Ibuprofen. This typical pain reliever comes from a family of medicines referred to as non-steroidal anti-inflammatory medicines (NSAIDs). They are readily available non-prescription (Advil, Motrin) and additionally by prescription. Heartburn, abdominal pain, as well as nausea, prevail adverse effects since these medicines aggravate the cellular lining of the stomach and oesophagus. Long-lasting usage can also lead to bleeding and stomach abscess. The most effective way to stay clear of these impacts is by adhering to the dosage directions on the packaging and by not taking these medicines on an empty tummy.

The "marvel medicine" is one more NSAID that can create heartburn as well as other digestive problems. Once more, most of these problems can be avoided by taking aspirin with food to help decrease its results on the oesophagus as well as tummy.

Iron supplements. This mineral can assist your body to make more red blood cells and battle iron-deficiency anaemia, however, it can additionally create acid reflux, indigestion, and also constipation. Try taking iron pills with food as well as prevent taking them at going to bed.

Hypertension medicines. Calcium network blockers such as nifedipine (Procardia) and also beta-blockers such as propranolol (Inderal) can additionally cause heartburn. Talk to your doctor if you have concerns. Most hypertension Dr.ugs are readily available and specific medications can also be as effective and can have fewer side effects.

Anti-anxiety medicines. Diazepam (Valium) or lorazepam (Ativan) can often create queasiness as well as heartburn. If your heartburn signs and symptoms linger, your physician will likely be able to suggest one more anti-anxiety medicine instead.

Tricyclic antifreeze. Tricyclic antidepressants that can produce acid reflux are the tricyclic antidepressants Amitriptyline (Vanatrip, Endep), Imitranil (Tofranil) and Nortriptyline (Pamelor, Aventyl). Ask your doctor if there may be fewer negative effects of a Dr.ug in a class of antidepressants.

Anti-biotics. The antibiotic tetracycline is used to treat microbial infections, consisting of pneumonia but can trigger looseness of the bowels, heartburn, and opposite effects.

If you presume that a medicine is triggering heartburn, don't stop taking you prescription Dr.ugs on your own. Call your doctor before you take the following dosage. Your clinical team might have the ability to make an alternative or recommend methods to stop heartburn symptoms. Occasionally, just transforming the moment of the day, you take your Dr.ug can help.

Treat the Burn With Heartburn Medicine

It is important to treat cardiovascular, especially if you have frequent symptoms. In fact, heartburn may damage your oesophagus over time. Talk to your doctor if prescription or non-prescription cardiovascular medicine is ideal for you.

There are many non-prescription heartburn medications offered:

Antacids like Mylanta or Maalox can counteract the results of stomach acid.

vH2 blockers such as ranitidine (Zantac), famotidine (Pepcid AC), and cimetidine (Tagamet) lowered stomach acid production.

Proton pump preventions such as omeprazole (Prilosec, Prilosec OTC) and also esomeprazole (Nexium) quit almost all acid manufacturing.

Making way of living modifications, including Dr.opping weight if you are obese, preventing late-night dishes, as well as giving up cigarette smoking may additionally assist put out the fire and alleviate your heartburn.

Iron, as well as potassium supplements, might also add to reflux. If you believe any of your medications are adding to reflux, talk to your physician. She or he might be able to recommend a choice without these negative effects.

STRESS

An often-cited Gallup survey found that almost two-thirds of heartburn patients said that their symptoms were worse. Absolutely nobody is why. Why does this happen? Professional people also assumed that depressed people could produce additional stomach acid, and some studies show that your feeling of reflux pain during periods of stress and fear increases.

Stress can also Dr.ive us toward other actions that can trigger heartburn, like smoking cigarettes, alcohol consumption alcohol, skipping the fitness centre, and also stress and anxiety eating. Chronic reflux itself might worsen stress.

Can Stress Cause Acid Reflux?

Do you find your signs and symptoms of heartburn or gastro oesophagus reflux disease (GERD) acting up at the worst times-- like throughout a job interview or right prior to your child's wedding celebration? Most individuals that experience heartburn could keep away from Uncle Ned's spicy chilli and also miss orange juice with breakfast. But they may be much less aware of how satisfying the moms and dads for the first time or providing a discussion might affect their symptoms.

According to some surveys and researches, stress and anxiety may extremely well be another trigger for heartburn. With some reliable coping methods, you can calm your stomach also throughout the most trying times.

The link

Lifestyle elements can contribute to how illness impacts an individual. A 2009 research study took a look at health surveys of over 40,000 Norwegians and located that people that reported work-related stress and anxiety were Dr.amatically much more in danger for GERD signs. People that stated they had reduced work satisfaction were two times as most likely to have GERD compared to those that reported high job contentment. a lot more recent research, published in Internal Medicine, interviewed 12,653 people with GERD and also discovered that nearly fifty per cent reported anxiety as the largest element that got worse signs and symptoms, also when on the Dr.ug.

Studies Showing a Link Between Anxiety as well as GERD

While anxiety is not listed as a root cause of GERD, a study published in 2013 showed the occurrence of anxiety in females with GERD is higher than for those in the general populace. People with both GERD and stress and anxiety might have much more constant signs and symptoms and more serious signs, leading to a lowered high quality of life.

Stress and anxiety might contribute to the development of GERD and in worsening of symptoms, although researchers aren't entirely clear how.

Some professionals believe that a mind chemical cholecystokinin (CCK), which has been linked to worry as well as food poisonings, might play a role in the frequency of GERD in individuals with stress and anxiety disorders. There are concepts that anxiousness can slow down digestion, rise stomach acid, or lead to enhanced muscle tension that can tax the belly.

One more possibility or adding factor might be that when individuals are anxious, they often tend to take part in behaviours that may intensify or cause heartburn, like smoking cigarettes, Dr.inking alcohol, or consuming deep-fried or fatty foods. These can be relaxing actions that can then lead to the pain as well as the pain of heartburn.

The same may also be accurate, because the GERD symptoms, such as upper body pain and swallowing difficulties, can cause concern and anxiety or an anxiety attack. It is important to remember that there is no cause in a web link.

A 2015 research study discovered that stress and anxiety and anxiety enhance the danger of GERD, and also various other studies have actually found that GERD's adverse effect on lifestyle raises anxiety and clinical depression, creating a vicious circle. Yet there is no scientific proof that favourably links stress and anxiety to enhanced belly acid.

A couple of researches, including a current study published in the clinical journal Gastroenterology, shows that lots of people with anxiety and also GERD signs, have regular oesophagus acid levels.

A number of researches have actually discovered that stress and anxiety appear to boost symptoms connected with GERD, such as heartburn and upper stomach discomfort. It's thought that stress and anxiety may make you much more sensitive to discomfort as well as other symptoms of GERD.

Anxiety, as well as various other mental distress, might also impact oesophagus mobility and the performance of your reduced oesophagus sphincter. Oesophagus mobility refers to the tightenings that happen in your oesophagus to relocate food toward your tummy.

Your reduced oesophagus sphincter is a ring of muscle around your lower oesophagus that relaxes to enable food and liquid right into your tummy and also closes to avoid the materials of your belly from flowing back up.

Does tension really make it worse?

It's still open to question whether stress, in fact, enhances the manufacturing of belly acid or literally creates a worsening in acid. Presently, several researchers think that when you're stressed, you come to be more sensitive to smaller sized amounts of acid in the oesophagus.

In 1993, scientists published in the American Journal of GastroenterologyTrusted Source that individuals with acid reflux who were anxious as well as emphasized reported having a lot more agonizing signs associated with acid reflux, yet no one showed a boost in gastric acid. Simply put, though people regularly reported feeling a lot more discomfort, the scientists really did not discover any type of boost incomplete acid generated.

One more research from 2008 included further support to this idea. They additionally located that it increased their symptoms by making them more sensitive to direct acid exposure when researchers subjected individuals with GERD to a difficult noise.

Is it all in your head?

Does this mean that the signs and symptoms are all in your head? Not likely. Researchers theorize that anxiety may trigger modifications in the brain that show up discomfort receptors, making you literally a lot more sensitive to minor increases in acid levels. Tension can likewise diminish the production of substances called prostaglandins, which usually protect the tummy from the results of acid. This could boost your assumption of pain.

Stress, combined with fatigue, might offer even more body modifications that cause boosted indigestion. Regardless of exactly what happens in the body and the mind, those who experience signs of indigestion know that stress and anxiety can make them feel uncomfortable, and also dealing with the way of living aspects is necessary.

Job Stress Brings Gastrointestinal Problems

Anxiety can be difficult on your gut. And that might be particularly true when the work environment is very demanding-- such as tidying up after the 9/11 attacks or offer in the army, according to researchers that have found a link in between these demanding tasks and also stomach problems.

The research studies existed this week at the yearly meeting of the American College of Gastroenterology in San Diego.

Workers who helped clean up the World Trade Center after the 9/11 attacks are more likely than the basic population to obtain GERD (gastro oesophagus reflux disease) in which belly materials return to the oesophagus, says Yvette Lam, MD, a gastroenterologist at Stony Brook University Medical Center, N.Y., who presented the results of the research at the conference.

She additionally discovered an association between GERD and psychological health disorders.

With her coworkers, she evaluated 697 people, ages 34 to 50, that helped with the clean-up. At the first visit, carried out in between October 2005 and also September 2006, 41% had GERD actually, compared to about 20% of the general population.

Researchers were also more likely to have conditions of mental health such as clinical depression or anxiety in those with GERD. 21 per cent of GERD suffering from post-traumatic stress disorder (PTSD) at first sight, 21.5 per cent were depressed, and nearly 30% were anxiety disorders.

In all, 413 clients came for the 2nd browse through carried out concerning two years later, to see if the problems lingered. the psychological illness continued, with 21.3% of those that had GERD at the initial go-to reporting PTSD and 32.8% coverage clinical depression.

" The GERD prevalence additionally rose with an increasing number of mental wellness disorders," Lam says. Weight problems, taken into consideration a danger element for GERD, had not been related to it in this study. But exposure to such points as dealing with human remains was connected with both the GERD as well as the PTSD, she says.

Therapy of the mental health conditions might be crucial to resolving the GERD, Lam says.

Gastrointestinal Problems in the Military

Gastrointestinal troubles are additionally common in army employees, says Mark Riddle, MD, Dr.PH, a researcher at the Naval Medical Research Center in Silver Spring, Md. Servicemen and also servicewomen, he says, "are under a lot of stress and anxiety as you can think of throughout deployment."

Riddle states the 4th leading root cause of sees to VA Medical Centers is gastrointestinal disorders.

To discover more, Riddle and his coworkers reviewed data from the Defense Medical Surveillance System, identifying nearly 32,000 situations of stomach problems in active service U.S. army personnel in between 1999 and also 2007. Among the troubles were irregular bowel movements, diarrhoea, cranky bowel disorder (IBS), and acid indigestion after an infection of the tummy as well as intestines (gastroenteritis).

When Riddle sought links in between the past stomach troubles as well as current ones, he discovered an organization between background of gastroenteritis-- an infection of the stomach and also intestinal tracts caused by germs, virus, or various other organisms-- as well as all sorts of intestinal issues later on.

The greatest danger was for looseness of the bowels as well as IBS. Having a history of gastroenteritis boosted the risk of looseness of the bowels sixfold, and of IBS nearly fourfold. The enhanced threat for irregularity or indigestion was much less, each about twofold.

The stomach troubles persist, Riddle discovered. Virtually 30% of the armed forces with issues were still getting care two years after the diagnosis.

The common advice to prevent intestinal infections-- such as boiling water or peeling off food that might be infected-- does not hold up in battle circumstances or emergency atmospheres such as the article 9/11 clean-up, Riddle says.

" We are developing vaccines to with any luck protect against [gastrointestinal infections]," he states.

" We require to come up I believe with a vaccination-- a great solution-- or chemoprophylaxis like you consider jungle fever. However, it would certainly need to be something you can securely consider a long period of time."

Although scientists don't yet totally recognize the connection between GERD and anxiousness, it's understood that anxiousness and also anxiety can cause or intensify signs related to GERD.

You might be able to soothe most of your symptoms of both conditions utilizing at-home treatments, but both conditions do warrant a visit to a doctor. Treatments are readily available that can assist you in handling or avoiding both problems.

GERD and also anxiety can both create upper body discomfort, which is additionally a sign of a heart attack. Get emergency situation medical care for any kind of brand-new chest pain, specifically if you also have a lack of breath, or arm or jaw pain.

SCLERODERMA

Lots of people with scleroderma list acid reflux as a symptom. Various other gastrointestinal signs in individuals with scleroderma include irregular bowel movements as well as diarrhoea.

Scleroderma is an autoimmune illness that triggers the skin, as well as sometimes other organs of the body, to become thick as well as difficult. In the scattered form of scleroderma, the oesophagus and gastrointestinal tract are frequently affected. GERD, or gastro oesophagus reflux illness, is a problem in which acid in the tummy streams backwards up into the oesophagus, causing heartburn and also other problems.

People with scleroderma commonly have GERD. The concern, obviously, is why.

How Scleroderma Causes GERD Symptoms

With scleroderma, the body immune system provokes the body right into producing too much collagen, the key protein discovered in connective cells. This added collagen gets transferred within the skin, making it hard. It can also get transferred in the organs, including the muscle mass of the oesophagus and digestive walls.

When the valve that maintains stomach acid from getting away up right into the oesophagus isn't working well, reflux takes place. That shutoff is called the lower oesophagus sphincter.

There are subtypes of scleroderma. A lot more restricted types influence just skin, while other types assault muscular tissue, lungs, heart, joints, as well as kidneys. When the muscular tissues of the gastrointestinal system are entailed, the oesophagus may be hit the hardest.

" Patients with scleroderma can have extremely severe GERD as a result of the involvement of the smooth muscle mass in the [reduced] two-thirds of the oesophagus, consisting of the reduced oesophagus sphincter," states gastroenterologist Lauren B. Gerson, MD, associate professor of medicine at Stanford University in Palo Alto, Calif

. In people with innovative scleroderma, the reduced component of the oesophagus, including the area around the lower oesophagus sphincter, can become hardened as well as thickened by scleroderma and is less able to operate generally. It can no longer smoothly push food downward right into the belly, and also the reduced oesophagus sphincter can no longer close tightly sufficient to keep acid in the tummy, where it belongs.

A gastroenterologist can do examinations that will certainly assist the patient and also physician discover how well the oesophagus is functioning. While scleroderma individuals usually have a rheumatologist looking after their overall problem, they also have to see several specialists, such as gastroenterologists, to look after specific elements of their wellness.

Dealing With GERD in Scleroderma Patients

Life with scleroderma can be really hard, yet there are medications that can alleviate GERD, decrease these undesirable signs and symptoms, and safeguard your oesophagus from the damage of repeated exposure to tummy acid.

" Patients frequently call for anti-reflux Dr.ug along with pro- [activity] agents," states Dr. Gerson. These two kinds of medications assist in maintain acid firmly below the reduced oesophagus sphincter, and also aid relocates food quickly down right into the stomach, to ensure that the reduced oesophagus sphincter doesn't obtain extended open for long term durations.

You need to likewise speak to your gastroenterologist concerning whether changing your diet might aid, as some sorts of food and Dr.ink have a tendency to cause more reflux.

You may intend to try the complying with approaches to restrict acid reflux right into the oesophagus:

Consume tiny meals more often, rather than 2 or three big meals that distend the stomach.

Keep upright for one to two hrs after consuming. Do not eat right before going to bed, for example, or late in the evening. This makes it more probable that acid will stay down in your stomach.

Raise your bedhead to make sure you rest at an angle.

Prevent spicy or fatty foods, high levels of caffeine as well as alcohol-- and any kind of other food that shows up to set off even more acid for you.

There is no remedy for scleroderma-- only treatments that can take care of signs and symptoms. GERD signs and symptoms usually respond well to treatment, so do not be reluctant to seek out a gastroenterologist if you have reflux or heartburn along with scleroderma.

The exact same basic techniques to reduce reflux can assist scleroderma people also: Avoid trigger foods as well as alcohol, don't lie down after consuming, eat smaller meals, as well as lose weight if you require to. Over-the-counter antacids may also help, yet talk to your medical professional before utilizing them.

ACID REFLUX SYMPTOMS (GERD)

Consistent heartburn is the most usual symptom of GERD.

Heartburn is a burning discomfort in the facility of the breast, behind the breastbone. It commonly begins in the upper abdomen as well as spreads out up right into the neck or throat.

The pain can last as long as 2 hrs.

Heartburn is normally even worse after consuming.

Lying down or flexing over can bring on heartburn or make it worse.

The discomfort generally does not start or become worse with physical activity.

Heartburn is often described as acid indigestion.

Not everyone with GERD has heartburn.

The pain and burning of the breast or throat that was named cardiovascular by the United States National Library of Medicine because of the belly acid backup right in your oesophagus

More than 60 million Americans experience something each month, which the American College of

Gastroenterology reports to 15 million Americans daily.

Would it certainly be very easy to detect such discomfort in your high body? Not exactly-heartburn signs and symptoms are sometimes less evident or misinterpreted.

Left untreated heartburn may lead to major issues, such as, for example, Timothy Pfanner, MD at College Station, as Assistant Professor of Internal Medicine noted Barrett's oesophagus, which prevails over cancer cells in Texas A&M Health Science Centre.

That's why it's important to get a heartburn medical diagnosis from the organization and then deal with it, with the aid of your doctor. So, to get the ball rolling, here are TK signs and symptoms — both normal and not-so-ordinary — that could mean that you have acid reflux.

Here are some symptoms-- both uncommon as well as usual-- that can indicate you have indigestion.

Symptoms Of GERD Consist Of:

- **You have sharp chest discomfort**

Plainly, upper body discomfort is a telltale sign of heartburn-- yet it can also be a sign of a heart attack.

Lots of individuals mistake heartburn for a heart attack. While you absolutely shouldn't identify yourself, there are a few means to tell if your chest pain is a cardiac arrest or heartburn relevant.

As an example, pain may feel extra as an impairment or stress in your breast in the heart-related upper body and may spread to the back, neck, jaw or arms. It is typically often related to suddenness, heat, nausea, difficulty breathing, or irregular pulses. In contrast, heart-brûling chest pain is generally harder, caused by fatty or Spicy Food and prepared changes (such as sitting or bending over). The pain of the chest can be intensified through consumption.

Still, if you're having chest pain and your' e stressed, get in touch with your physician simply to rule out a cardiac arrest, claims Walter J. Coyle, MD, gastroenterologist with Scripps Clinic Torrey Pines in La Jolla, California.

- **When you lie down, your discomfort is worse**

Your signs can aggravate when you lie down or bend over because heartburn is created by tummy acid that sneaks back into your oesophagus. "If you're sitting up directly, gravity assists keep food in the belly," claims Dr. Coyle. "If you lose gravity, you're much more susceptible to reflux."

A quick solution? Most people with chronic heartburn usually raise their heads so that they do not lie horizontally entirely. If you have heartburn, it is also important to avoid eating meals before you go to bed.

- **You have pain after consuming**

The discomfort that sets in right after a dish-- specifically a big meal-- typically implies the stomach is strained and also its materials have no place to go but up. The good news is, there's a quick solution: "I would certainly emphasize not consuming large, fatty meals and watching [your intake of alcohol as well as tobacco]," claims Dr. Coyle, who is a spokesperson for the American College of Gastroenterology. (FYI: It's additionally another reason not to dine-then-recline.).

- **You have a bitter preference in your mouth**

Sometimes acid getting away from your belly can make its way right into the back of your throat, leaving a disgusting, bitter preference in your mouth. In really extreme situations, this can create choking, if that takes place-- particularly at night-- you should see a doctor. "I'm really aggressive with treatment if patients wake up choking," says Dr. Coyle, adding that he usually suggests acid-suppressing medicines like proton pump preventions, H2 blockers, Just as well as the antacids. (Dr. Coyle is in the Chair of the Takeda Pharmaceuticals Office, which markets the prevention of proton pumps).

- **You sound like you have a cool**

You might presume that when your voice starts cracking, you start to feel cold. Nevertheless, heartburn and symptoms can be additional.

If belly acid is leaking into your oesophagus, it can aggravate your vocal cables, claims Dr. Pfanner, that is also a gastroenterologist at Scott & White, in Temple, Texas. When your voice seems huskier than typical, pay attention to. You may have reflux if it's after you've consumed.

- **Your throat aches**

A sore throat is another timeless cool or flu symptom that might actually be caused by digestive issues.

You may have heartburn if your throat often tends to hurt only after meals. Nevertheless, as opposed to cold or flu, this kind of aching throat can also be constant. If you do not show any other signs, such as sneezing or sniffing, think about indigestion.

- **You have a nagging coughing**

For addition, other respiratory problems, such as constant resistance and hissing, can be due to heartburn, possibly because your lungs get stomach acid.

If you presume heartburn is at the origin of your breathing problems-- possibly due to the fact that it occurs right away after consuming-- you may wish to talk to your doctor about obtaining a pH examination. If you have acid reflux, the test is an outpatient procedure that determines the amount of acid in your oesophagus over a 24-hour period and also can help figure out.

- **Your asthma gets triggered-- commonly**

Coughing and wheezing from heartburn can get so severe that it can give rise to asthma. It is not clear, however, whether chronic heartburn actually causes bronchial asthma to develop in individuals. Although many individuals who have heartburn have asthma as well as the other way around, the overlapping factors are not clear.

Specialists believe tummy acid can activate nerves in the breast to constrict your breathing tubes in order to maintain acid from going into. Once more, a simple pH test to seek acid in your oesophagus might aid you to obtain to the bottom of the trouble.

- **You really feel nauseous after dishes frequently**

Queasiness has many issues that it can be difficult to connect to reflux. Dr. Coyle notes, "the only symptom they have of reflux in certain cases is diarrhoea. If you have queasiness, you can't figure out why there's reflux."

And if after dinner the queasiness goes forward, it is much more of an indication that acid reflux will occur. A routine anti-acid treatment like an anti-acid medicine may decrease your discomfort.

- **Your mouth fills with saliva suddenly**

If your mouth suddenly starts producing additional saliva, it could be water brash, which is very symptomatic of heartburn, Dr. Coyle claims.

It includes the very same nerves and also reflex as when you throw up. "Your body is trying to wash out an irritant in your oesophagus.

- **You have trouble ingesting**

Dr. Pfanner believes that in time the constant cycle of harm and cure after heartburn causes scarring. As a result, the lower oesophagus is swollen, causing the oesophagus to become compressed and the difficulty to swallow.

Various other signs and symptoms of GERD include:

- Regurgitation of bitter acid up right into the throat while bending or sleeping over.
- Bitter preference in the mouth.
- Persistent Dr.y coughing.
- Hoarseness (especially in the morning)
- Feeling of tightness in the throat, as if an item of food is stuck there.
- Trouble ingesting.
- Sore throat.
- Wheezing.
- Nausea.
- Post-meal discomfort in the abdomen.

One of the most typical symptoms in infants as well as kids is repeated vomiting, coughing, and also various other respiratory issues.

Reasons Not To Ignore Gerd Symptoms

Unattended gastro oesophagus reflux disease (GERD) can cause a range of illness

A burning problem

For many Americans, heartburn is just periodic trouble. Sixty million individuals get it a minimum of when a month.

For the 19 million individuals that have a persistent form of heartburn understood as gastro oesophagus reflux illness (GERD), without treatment,signs and symptoms can lead to a range of wellness complications.

If you experience prolonged or frequent heartburn (twice a week regularly), see your physician.

GERD isn't hazardous or deadly in itself. Long-lasting GERD can lead to extra significant health and wellness troubles.

Esophagitis: Esophagitis is the irritation as well as swelling the stomach acid causes in the cellular lining of the oesophagus. Esophagitis can create abscess in your oesophagus, heartburn, and upper body bleeding, pain and also problem swallowing.

In GERD, food, acid, and also digestive system juices recede into the oesophagus, the tube that connects the throat to the tummy. With time, this causes inflammation as well as swelling, called esophagitis.

"If you've had direct exposure to your oesophagus for only several weeks, you can develop a lining of inflammation," said Anish Sheth, MD, an Assistant Professor of Digestive System Disease at the Yale School of Medicine, New Haven Conn.

Oesophagus stricture

Mark tissue can tighten the oesophagus if esophagitis goes on also long Called a stricture, this can make it difficult or painful to ingest.

Big pieces of food can obtain stuck as well as may call for an endoscopy to remove them. You may likewise go to threat of choking, and you can lose excess weight if you prevent food and also beverages due to a stricture.

An expansion or expansion of the oesophagus is treated with stringency. It may need to be multiplied. Nonetheless, medications such as proton pump inhibitors (PPIs, for example) may avoid acid-blocking. It may not return.

Barrett's oesophagus

If left without treatment for many years, consistent indigestion can cause precancerous adjustments in cells; a problem called Barrett's oesophagus. The condition does not cause signs and symptoms, but a medical professional can detect it is by executing an endoscopy.

A tiny portion of individuals with Barrett's oesophagus develops oesophagus cancer, which is usually fatal.

"If you have heartburn for more than twice a week or if you have signs and symptoms that are worsening or have no new ones, those are all reasons to have a look," says Dr. Sheth.

Throat and voice troubles

The main GERD sign is heartburn, but not all individuals obtain it. They might have other, harder-to-diagnose signs and symptoms.

" We call them instances of 'quiet reflux,'" says Dr. Sheth. "The client may not have heartburn as it's classically explained. However, they can have a selection of other issues that are taking place outside of the oesophagus-- like hoarseness, voice changes, sore throat, or chronic cough. They have this feeling that there's a lump in their throat, or that they frequently have to remove their throat."

Breathing troubles

If tummy acid is respired after it is revitalised, GERD can aggravate bronchial asthma or pneumonia. GERD can cause shortness of breath and difficulty breathing even without lung problems.

A double-edged sword maybe therapy. According to several reports, GERD medicines such as PPIs may indeed increase the risk of pneumonia. (They can promote bacterial growth, hypothesize researchers, or reduce the coughing that can help the lung to be removed).

Deal with your doctor, that may take into consideration lung feature when dealing with reflux.

Dental cavity

When belly acid as well as digestion juices make their back up the oesophagus and also right into the mouth, it can create a sour taste and also, if it occurs regularly sufficient, wear off tooth enamel and promote dental caries.

People with acid-reflux-induced erosion are typically not aware of the damage until it gets to an innovative phase.

In a University of Alabama research, 40% of GERD patients had substantial dental caries (as did 70% of those whose reflux reached the top oesophagus), contrasted to only 10% of those without any reflux.

Oesophagus ulcers

Tummy acid can wear away the oesophagus cellular lining, creating abscess or sores. Individuals with ulcers might spit up or vomit blood, or see it in the stool.

Tell your doctor immediately if you have such signs. An endoscopy–a long and versatile pipe in the mouth to examine the GI tract–can detect oesophagus ulcers and acid-blocking or acid-reduction meds.

Oesophagal cancer cells

In really severe cases, unattended GERD (and subsequent Barrett's oesophagus) can lead to cancer of the oesophagus. In 2010, 16,640 new instances of oesophagal cancer were diagnosed in the U.S. The major threat aspects are smoking cigarettes, Dr.inking alcohol, poor diet plan, and persistent reflux illness.

Signs include weight loss, problem ingesting, or stomach blood loss claims Dr. Sheth. "It's something that occurs over years of reflux damages, so for someone who's 30 and also or else healthy and balanced, we probably will not take into consideration cancer," states Dr. Sheth. "But if you're over 50 and you've had heartburn for years and also you're suddenly slimming down, for instance, it's certainly something we intend to evaluate for.".

Lower quality of life

In addition to health dangers, GERD signs can influence a person's health and wellness and joy.

In a 2003 German study of more than 6,000 GERD individuals, many reported that their lifestyle had actually been endangered due to issues with sleep, food, and beverage, along with social and also physical limitations. (There are also financial consequences as a result of buying numerous heartburn medications.).

Quality of life for the GERD clients resembled heart-attack individuals, and also sometimes, also lower than those for cancer and diabetes mellitus.

CAN GERD (CHRONIC INDIGESTION) TRIGGER ASTHMA?

We don't understand the specific connection between GERD as well as asthma. Greater than 75% of people with asthma have GERD. They are two times as most likely to have GERD as individuals without bronchial asthma. GERD may make asthma signs and symptoms worse, and bronchial asthma Dr.ugs may make GERD worse. Dealing with GERD frequently assists in easing bronchial asthma symptoms.

The symptoms of GERD can hurt the lining of the throat, lungs and also respiratory tracts, making breathing difficult and also causing relentless coughing, which may recommend a link. Physicians mainly check out GERD as a source of asthma if:

- Bronchial asthma begins in their adult years.
- Asthma symptoms get worse after a dish, workout, during the night as well as after relaxing.

- Bronchial asthma does not improve with standard asthma therapies.
- If you have bronchial asthma and also GERD, your doctor can aid you to discover the most effective ways to handles both conditions-- the best medications and treatments that will not exacerbate signs of either condition.

TREATMENT OPTIONS FOR ACID REFLUX

Choosing a Natural Treatment for GERD or GERD Mediations?

Finding a heartburn therapy or a natural treatment for GERD is in fact rather basic, as well as you don't automatically have to go the clinical route with indigestion Dr.ug if you are seeking acid reflux soothes.

There are all-natural cures for acid reflux, a diet plan for indigestion, natural heartburn treatments, a heartburn pillow, as well as even natural home remedy for indigestion.

The GERD diet is really one of the very best GERD treatment choices, specifically if you are eliminating all the heartburn food to stay clear of.

Medication, also surgery, may be needed, particularly you have serious GERD symptoms, yet lots of people feel extra comfy without medication in their bodies, and ideally, an all-natural remedy for GERD and a natural heartburn treatment is excellent an excellent place to begin.

I indicate, if you can go the natural path, why not attempt!

WHAT DOES ACID REFLUX (GERD) FEEL LIKE?

Acid reflux typically feels like a painful or shedding feeling in your tummy, upper abdomen behind the breastbone, oesophagus, and also equalize right into your throat. You might have the feeling of a warm, acidic, or sour-tasting liquid at the rear of the throat or an aching throat.

It might feel like it's difficult to swallow or really feel rigidity in the throat when you have heartburn, and also it might feel as if food is embedded your throat or oesophagus.

When you relax, bend over or after eating, you may have chest pain. (See your medical practitioner for any undiagnosed chest pain, presume you do not have heartburn until you are identified by a medical practitioner).

UX (GERD) DIET

A GERD diet plan is a vital part of the treatment for both occasional heartburn, also referred to as acid reflux, and also gastro oesophagus reflux condition, which is a much more chronic problem. The diet concentrates on eliminating foods that decrease lower oesophagal sphincter (LES) stress, hold-up stomach emptying, and raise belly acid, every one of which raises your threat of belly acid streaming right into your oesophagus.

GERD's Diet plan does not fit into all of the sizes, so it is very important that you try out the diet in order to recognize and remove foods that cause your upper body or throat to burn.

Exactly how It Works

The GERD diet regimen aids you to:

- Stay away from foods and beverages that worsen heartburn

- Select extra foods that can assist control tummy acid manufacturing
- Develop eating routines that can decrease your signs and symptoms
- Include a well-balanced selection of nutrient-dense and also healthy foods that will certainly aid you to keep a healthy and balanced weight

This is mainly attained through food options, though meal size and timing does figure in.

If you have chronic GERD and get heartburn regularly, you can gain from the GERD diet regimen by following it long-term. Even if you experience signs infrequently, ending up being accustomed to as well as maintaining a close eye on the usage of trigger foods may assist you in protecting against symptoms.

Foods to consume on an acid spectator diet plan

Food is just one of the best happiness in life, but as everyone has actually experienced at once or another, eating specific foods can bring pain. This is specifically true if you're delicate to particular active ingredients, textures or flavours, or tend to consume incredibly rapidly. A food-related discomfort that's particularly aggravating (and can be painful) is indigestion, or heartburn, which emerges (cough) when food isn't digested well. Eating foods as well as Dr.inks that protect against heartburn can assist reduce the opportunities of heartburn, indigestion, pain, nausea or vomiting, and enhance the opportunities you obtain the most out of what you eat.

" Acid reflux takes place when there is a weakening in the sphincter between your oesophagus and also tummy," Samantha Cochrane, a registered dietitian at The Ohio State University Wexner Medical Center, informs Bustle. Points like hormonal adjustments, smoking, certain medications, and certain foods can lead to acid reflux, Cochrane states.

As a certified health and wellness train, I deal with customers on having healthy and balanced food digestion, and also with this, we generally review eating slower in order to be more mindful as well as to alleviate the gastrointestinal process, without overwhelming the body with large quantities of protein, acid, and also various other substances that your gastrointestinal system then has to pass. Such can delay the digestion procedure and cause signs and symptoms of heartburn, such as heartburn as well as acid indigestion, in addition to a bad taste in the mouth, trouble breathing, and scratchiness.

Heartburn really is just gastro oesophagus reflux (GERD) term or short heartburn. Matthew Bechtold, a gastroenterologist at the University of Missouri Health Care, says indigestion is "heartburn" because it essentially feels like your chest is on fire. "Heartburn is the term used by people because they feel a burning sensation in the breast, but it is truly indigestion coming from your stomach and creating pain," he explains.

This is not only a burning sight, however. Individuals with acid reflux may, according to Dr. Bechtold:

Feel like food is coming back up right into their throat;

Have chronic coughing, specifically at night when they're laying down a level;

Or have problem ingesting as a result of swelling in the oesophagus.

There are a few explanations of why this is happening. Dr. Bechtold argues that certain foods can relax the lower oesophagus and allow reflux to be restored directly into the oesophagus. Those foods are a tuffet he calls the "3 great sins": "caffeine, chocolate and alcohol–specifically merlot–are sure to all relax low oesophagus muscles and allow acid to come back," he describes and adds that such acidic foods and foods as spicy ones are spicy. They are also known to the Providence Saint John's Health Centre in Santa Monica.

Thankfully, there are likewise foods to assist you battle heartburn by either preventing it or helping to relieve it

While avoiding foods that create heartburn isn't always possible-- imagine Sunday suppers without meatballs and also pasta, as an example-- it's worth keeping this listing in the back of your mind for times you especially wish to prevent indigestion.

Here are foods and Dr.inks that can help prevent acid reflux.

1. Bananas & Melon

Generally, the name of the game in regards to consuming to stay clear of heartburn will be to consume low-acid food and Dr.inks-- which consists of fruit. Preventing citrus or other acidic fruit container aid avoid indigestion, according to the Cleveland Clinic. Bananas as well as melons, by comparison, are lower in acid, implying that they are much less likely to cause indigestion signs and symptoms, according to Dr. Jamie Koufman, who recommended these fruits to The New York Times.

2. Oatmeal

The traditional breakfast cereal has a pH of 7.2, says The New York Times, making it a really neutral enhancement to your day (no wordplay here meant). Oatmeal can go down really quickly and keep you going for hours to come. In fact, it can aid in many other digestive treatments, with one 2005 study searching for oatmeal to support chilDr.en with acid reflux poop easier.

3. Fruity/Flavored Gum

Gum tissue can be used in an unusual way to help treat heartburn; saliva production and low acid saliva are called for, and it is used to relieve the inflamed oesophagus, according to Harvard Health. Cochrane claims. However, that spirit or peppermint can trigger acid reflux, so it is much better to stick to the flavoured fruit-tissue of the gum or to a more neutral taste.

4. Ginger

The science on its results on heartburn is average: a 2019 review of ginger's impacts on digestion discovered that while ginger had a favourable internet effect on queasiness, one of its couple of, unusual side effects was actually heartburn. No matter, the research wrapped up that "ginger could be taken into consideration a harmless and perhaps efficient choice choice" for nausea or vomiting as well as various other digestive system concerns, and that even more research study is required, so if ginger assists you, more power to you.

➤ Health Benefits Of Ginger

In the kitchen, we've long utilized ginger-- in anything from ginger molasses cookies as well as ginger tea to Indian- and also Asian-inspired meals-- as a flavour-agent. Besides being one of the tastiest and most recognizable seasonings on the planet, ginger root has also been marketed for a long time as a cure for a variety of health and wellness issues. Today, the health and wellness benefits of ginger are coming to be extra recognized by both Western medicine experts and the wellness-minded among us with anecdotal evidence.

Nutritionally, the seasoning is a celebrity. In an entire cup of chopped fresh ginger root, you'll discover just around 80 calories, less than 18 grams of carbs, as well as concerning 2 grams of fibre and protein. Throw in a tablespoon to a recipe, and you're including much less than 5 calories, which is why Keri Gans, RDN, licensed yoga exercise trainer as well as owner of Keri Gans Nutrition, says, "ginger is utilized in such small amounts and is so reduced in calories that it doesn't ever use high amounts of calories, carbs, or sugar." Each zingy bite of ginger additionally includes minerals and vitamins like iron, vitamin C, potassium, magnesium, as well as zinc.

While the root itself may look daunting, don't let it be turned off; ginger is actually offered (as well as valuable) in a variety of forms. "Ginger may be used fresh, Dr.ied, powdered, peeled or as oil, chips or juice,"

Maybe the health benefits of ginger will if its flavour and nutrient account aren't enough to send you running to the farmers market or grocery shop. Read on to get more information concerning how ginger can increase your health.

* **Ginger can stop nausea**

Ever been informed to pop a ginger lozenge throughout an especially rough car and truck flight? Because ginger can help soothe an upset belly, that's. Research recommends ginger can remedy queasiness from travelling, pregnancy, or even radiation treatment, claims Julie Upton, RD, founder of Appetite for Health.

One Thai research located that ginger functioned as well as dimenhyDr.inate (the active ingredient in non-prescription motion-sickness medications) at dealing with as well as protecting against nausea or vomiting in pregnant ladies.

However, "since ginger has a lot of bioactive compounds, if you have clinical conditions or are expecting, you should inform your healthcare professional that you are taking ginger and how much," Upton claims.

- **It might decrease gas, irregularity, and also bloat**

Ginger might also relieve other GI concerns, many thanks to its digestive enzyme called zingibain that assists the body damage down healthy protein. The compound potentially aids the food you consume travel through your system more quickly-- and, subsequently, decreases the bloat, constipation, or gas you're experiencing.

But when you already seem like a flatterer fish, the last point you want to do is consume a square meal that happens to include the seasoning. Instead, appreciate a mug of homemade ginger tea-- made by soaking a couple of pieces of sliced ginger in a mug of warm water for five to 10 mins-- as well as Dr.ink it gradually. (Or try brand names like Yogi Ginger Tea as well as Traditional Medicinals Organic Ginger Aid.).

- What about ale of ginger? In most products, there is little or no true ginger, and there may be high fructose maize syrup, which can exacerbate the bloat. Before taking the course on soft Dr.inks, check the active ingredients and recommend Goose.

Ginger might aid fight infections

You might be turning to OJ when you really sense a chill coming on. Yet fresh ginger juice (or ginger smoothie) might make a much better choice, thanks to gingerol — an active ingredient — in ginger that might help you battle the virus. One laboratory research published in the Journal of Ethnopharmacology discovered that fresh ginger might be effective versus the human respiratory system syncytial virus (HRSV), a common cause of respiratory infections.

Well worth stating, the researchers discovered that Dr.ied out ginger was less effective than fresh ginger. Before you thoughtlessly acquire the origin, make certain you're selecting a chunk with smooth, unblemished skin. The more bark-like the root looks, the much less fresh it most likely is.

- **It may minimize menstrual aches**

Are you tormented by duration aches? Iranian research released in the Journal of Alternative and Complementary Medicine located that ginger was as reliable as ibuprofen for eliminating uncomfortable periods.

The research study individuals took a 250-milligram ginger powder capsule four times a day for 3 days as soon as they started their durations. You can likewise attempt soaking 2 tbsps of fresh ginger root in warm water, stressing, and enjoying with honey or lemon.

- **It fights to swell**

Gingerol is an antioxidant in ginger that might help reduce swelling, says Gans. Research recommends ginger extract supplements, as well as topical ginger lotion, may minimize tightness as well as pain in individuals with osteoarthritis (but deal with your health care company to create a thorough therapy prepare for any inflammatory problem).

Gym-fiends and also runners, this one's for you: A small study out of the University of Georgia located that everyday ginger supplements additionally minimized exercise-induced muscle pain.

- **Ginger may protect versus colon cancer**

One tiny research published in 2011 in Cancer Prevention Research suggested that ginger supplements might help prevent intestines cancer cells, specifically in those with an enhanced danger, thanks to its anti-inflammatory results on the gut. A lot more study is required to really understand this link, as well as it's worth noting that study participant took a huge dose of the spice (eight 250-milligram capsules a day).

- **it can assist weight management**

Natural herbs and flavours, in general, are beneficial for Dr.opping weight since the included flavours can aid you to feel much more completely satisfied with lower-calorie foods. Ginger's no various: One tiny research released in the journal Metabolism discovered that guys who consumed alcohol a warm ginger beverage (made from ginger powder and also hot water) after eating felt full for longer. "The results, showing boosted thermogenesis and also reduced sensations of hunger with ginger consumption, suggest a prospective role of ginger in weight monitoring," the scientists compose.

For a slender morning meal with a killer kick, try spraying ginger powder onto Greek yoghurt with berries.

5. Milk of Almond

According to Robynne Chutkan, a gastroenterologist in Washington, D.C., as well as the author of Gutbliss in an interview with Prevention, alcohol consumption of almond milk will reduce indigestion and help prevent it from occurring due to its vital nutrients and also the ability to alkalize the body and allow it to grow properly.

" Often cow's milk will lead to reflux, so almond milk is a great alternative, "said Beth Warren, MS, RDN, CDN, for a brief previous article on indigestion."Almond milk is alkaline-- the opposite of acidic-- helping to combat acid reflux." Dr.ink level or add to healthy smoothies after a meal.

- **Almonds as well as Acid Reflux**

If you have acid reflux, you can wonder if the almonds would improve or exacerbate the symptoms. Almonds are also low-acid foods that may play a role in the administration of an acid reflux sign. Inevitably, pay attention to your symptoms to decide how well this nutritious nut blends into your acid reflux diet plan.

Almonds as well as Acid Reflux

Heartburn occurs when the reduced oesophagal sphincter, situated on top of the tummy, does not close properly, and the belly components back up right into the oesophagus and throat. These swallow contents can be extremely acidic, and when spitting up, can trigger pain and pain. You might have heard that almonds can assist with acid reflux. While almonds have many health advantages, there is an absence of top-quality research specifically concerning almonds and acid reflux. Based on their nourishment account, almonds might have a positive effect on acid reflux illness.

> ➢ **Benefits of Almond Nutrition**

According to 2013 scientific guidelines released by the American College of Gastroenterology (ACG), slimming down is a key way of life technique to enhance or protect against acid reflux. A June 2014 review released in "The American Journal of Clinical Nutrition" wrapped up that despite their fat material, nuts might enhance weight management when part of a lowered calorie diet. Nuts aid regulates hunger, one of the reasons for this benefit, since calorie intake is lowered after consuming nuts. If a component of an effective weight loss plan, Eating a handful of almonds every day may indirectly assist acid reflux.

Almonds are a good resource of fibre, and according to a January 2005 research in "Gut," a diet plan high in fibre is linked to a lowered risk of indigestion symptoms. Eating foods high in fibre can also stop constipation. While this might not directly assist acid reflux signs and symptoms, fibre can help accomplish regular bowel movements, alleviating digestive symptoms such as bloating as well as abdominal pain.

➢ Benefits of Alkaline Almonds

Almonds, along with almond butter and also almond milk, are fairly alkaline foods, particularly when compared to higher acid foods such as tomatoes and also citrus fruits. Restricting these foods may benefit some acid reflux victims since acidic foods may aggravate the already irritated oesophagus. In addition, eating lower acid foods may lower the level of acidity of the stomach contents, so if reflux occurs, less irritation and also damage takes place. Top-quality research is not offered on the advantages of a low-acid diet in acid reflux administration. Some people may find symptom relief when they consume lower acid foods.

➢ Potential Problems

Because of an absence of research study revealing renovation in signs, ACG's medical standards do not advise the addition of details foods to assist acid reflux, neither do these guidelines support global evasion of usual trigger foods such as high or acidic fat foods. Consuming large quantities of almonds or almond butter right before bed can pose an issue-- nighttime acid reflux is a lot more most likely if you eat within two to three hrs of going to bed.

> **Warnings as well as Precautions**

Diet plan and way of living steps such as weight decrease may be the very first level of treatment to boost your indigestion. Additionally, acid-blocking medications are commonly utilized to take care of signs and symptoms. Past these essentials, with tracking your signs and symptoms, you might be able to determine foods that enhance or intensify your acid reflux. If you tolerate them as well as eat modest sections, almonds, as well as various other nuts, can be a healthy and balanced addition to your diet regimen. Nonetheless, tree nuts, consisting of almonds, are a typical root cause of food allergic reactions, which can bring about a fatal reaction. A slow-moving intro may be smart if almonds have actually not been a component of your diet in the past. Work with your medical professional on a monitoring strategy if your reflux signs and symptoms are regular or extreme. Heartburn can bring about serious health issue if neglected.

6. Greek Yogurt

Greek yoghurt, skyr, or kefir which have pressures of healthy and balanced gut promoting bacteria and probiotic homes, have actually been revealed to aid stop heartburn.

" Foods with healthy and balanced bacteria [such as yoghurt] might assist improve digestion as well as reduce the regularity of acid reflux," nutritionist Lisa Hugh previously told Bustle. Have yoghurt for breakfast or snack. It's additionally loaded with various other essential nutrients and also protein.

If you have acid reflux, you may ask yourself if alcohol consumption milk as well as eating yoghurt will certainly make your symptoms even worse. While specific foods are typically considered triggers of acid reflux, the American College of Gastroenterology's 2013 medical technique guidelines outline that there is not sufficient proof to support blanket food constraints in acid reflux monitoring.

- **Milk and also Reflux**

If high-fat foods worsen reflux, low-fat or nonfat milk might be much better tolerated compared to entire milk. If chocolate makes your reflux symptoms even worse, white milk may be better tolerated than chocolate milk. While lactose intolerance is not connected to acid reflux, individuals can endure from both conditions, as well as eliminating the angering foods can assist handle symptoms.

- **Yoghurt and Acid Reflux**

In basic, yoghurt is well tolerated as well as does not aggravate acid reflux symptoms. The quality study is lacking, and there is initial information recommending that probiotics might enhance acid reflux signs and symptoms. Since this study was not concentrated on acid reflux, more research study is required to make clear if probiotic-rich yoghurt or probiotics in basic help acid reflux management.

- **Cow's Milk Allergy and also Acid Reflux**

According to the August 2011 problem of "Gut as well as Liver," some types of serious heartburn have been related to cow's milk allergic reaction in chilDr.en. According to this write-up, a medical diagnosis of cow's milk allergic reaction was thought about in one-third of the pediatric situations with signs and symptoms of indigestion condition. The writers sum up that cow's milk allergic reaction can mimic or worsen the symptoms and signs of serious indigestion in infancy. This research study was finished on kids under the age of 2, so extra research study is needed to determine if this also relates to adults.

7. Liquorice

Similar to ginger, liquorice is a long-touted organic treatment for heartburn. A 2014 testimonial of case reports found that degly-cyrrhizinated liquorice aided youngsters to take care of acid reflux as a component of a more comprehensive integrative therapy.

8. Fennel

If you don't like the taste of liquorice, you probably won't like the preference of fennel, either, but recognize that both of these bitterly beautiful herbs can help with heartburn, according to Providence St. Joseph's Health. Fennel has a strong ability to help relieve the stomach and also the digestive system and to minimize the acidity. For best results, eat fennel as part of a salad or after a meal.

- **Fennel Seeds for Treatment of Heartburn**

Fennel is a perennial plant with enjoyable smelling bright yellow blossoms. It is native to Mediterranean areas however is found around the globe.

Its seeds are utilized for edible functions in addition to for medical reasons. Dr.ied seeds of fennel are made use of to make tea, oil, and also medicines.

It tastes and looks comparable to that of anise yet is not to be puzzled with it.

It also shares comparable medical residential or commercial properties with anise seeds as well as is utilized to treat different intestinal system conditions such as heartburn, colic, indigestion, cholera in addition to others such as coughs, respiratory issues, respiratory disease, backache, and visual problems.

Fennel oil is made use of in food and also in specific laxatives as a flavouring agent, and also as a fragrance element in soaps as well as packaged food products.

It is additionally sometimes utilized as a plaster for serpent attacks. Fennel is claimed to have an antispasmodic effect on the muscles, which is mostly a reason it relieves heartburn and various other belly troubles.

Nonetheless, it additionally has several various other buildings which add up to its medicinal results on the intestine.

1. Fennel helps Treats Stomach Spasms

When given up higher concentrations, fennel seeds work as anti uncertain for the belly. Stomach muscle spasms are just one of the major sources of discomfort in the upper body as a result of heartburn.

When the acid gets in touches with the walls of the gullet and damages them, the nerve signals initiate spasmolytic activity in the digestive tract as well as trigger the burning sensation and also discomfort.

Fennel seeds have been revealed to relax the tummy of the tummy as well as hinder the convulsions, therefore decreasing the discomfort caused by acid reflux.

The major components of fennel and also majorly fennel oil has been found to be Cis-panthenol as well as fenchone.

Both these compounds are responsible for the particular scent of fennel and also for its antispasmodic impact.

These phenolic compounds are antinociceptive in nature which indicates that they decrease the level of sensitivity towards discomfort stimuli.

This is meant to be the predominant reason for the capability of fennel to reduce pains.

A stomach discomfort in infants is called colic and is a significant reason for childish pain.

The only medicine readily available for colic in infants is dicyclomine hyDr.ochloride which often has actually been revealed to apply serious adverse effects on the newly born.

Fennel seed tea has actually been revealed to be very efficient in dealing with infantile colic by loosening up the convulsions created in the tummy.

2. Fennel seeds show a Carminative Effect on the Gut

Gas or windiness is uncomfortable by item of heartburn created because of indigestion.

Fennel seed teas as well as products have actually been located to be extremely effective for soothing windiness and enhancing digestion.

This more stops the approaching pain assaults due to the motion of gas in the stomach.

These carminative results of fennel are credited to the odorant substances found in the seeds which have high medical residential or commercial properties.

3. Fennel seeds Enhance Gastro-oesophagus Motility

Acid indigestion and also consequent heartburn is sometimes advertised by reduced gastro-oesophagus mobility.

The food, as well as the stomach acids, are not able to pass down as a result of much less motile tract and create pain.

Fennel seeds have actually been revealed to enhance the gastro-oesophagus motility which helps press food downwards appropriately to make sure that acid indigestion, as well as acid reflux, is stopped, thus amelioration the discomfort.

4. Anti-inflammatory and also anti-oxidative results of fennel seeds

Oxidation and also inflammation are necessary repercussions of heartburn which intensify the discomfort as well as a result in an ulcer, gut wall surface damage as well as also cancers.

The heartburn reveals the walls of the gullet to the strong acid of the belly that erodes its safety mucous layer.

This erosion leads to the activation of particular immune facilities that generate inflammation.

The damage to the intestine wall additionally triggers the responsive oxygen varieties or oxygen radicals that attack the healthy cells as well as cause further damages.

Fennel seed oil or fennel seed alcoholic extract has been revealed to apply both anti-oxidative and anti-inflammatory effect on experimental subjects.

It has strengthening been reported that fennel seeds boost the activity of glutathione, a compound that actively scavenges the oxygen radicals.

It likewise has the capacity to minimize the task of peroxidases that promote the manufacturing of responsive oxygen species.

Likewise, fennel crucial oils have a substance called pinene, which helps in minimizing the inflammation by blocking the inflammatory immune pathway in the tummy.

It additionally lowers the task of a professional inflammatory cytokine IL-8 in a focus reliant manner.

- **Dose and Consumption**

Fennel seeds are normally considered risk-free to eat after dishes or as edibles in dishes. Fennel preparations, teas and also oils are commonly utilized to minimize belly troubles and various other disorders.

The most typical dose of fennel to avoid stomach problems consisting of heartburn is chewing half a teaspoon of Dr.ied seeds after each meal or more frequently.

There is insufficient evidence for the optimum dosage and also adverse effects which is why it is suggested to maintain the dosage low.

Fennel tea products can be prepared by steaming concerning half a tsp (about 3 grams) in water for 15 mins, cooling, straining and also consuming the exact same 2-3 times a day.

Again, very little study has actually been done on the safety of the tea so the dosage needs to be kept a minimum of a doctor must be asked for suggestions.

Fennel oil is readily available out there and also needs to be taken as routed on the label.

9. Lean Protein

While the food that has a greater fat content isn't necessarily "poor" for you-- avocados, as an example, are chock-full of it-- fat can aggravate heartburn. "Choosing lean, healthy protein resources such as lean meats, fish, beans, vegetables, and low-fat dairy can aid stop reflux when a replacement for proteins higher in fat," Cochrane claims.

10. Aloe

You might think of aloe vera as a gel that you use to treat sunburn, but the anti-inflammatory results that make it a calming post-vacation skin treatment make the plant effective when treating acid reflux. A randomized control study released in 2015 found that it was "risk-free and well-tolerated and also reduced the regularity of all GERD signs and symptoms assessed." You can choose it as juice from most grocery stores.

Aloe vera is a succulent plant frequently found in exotic environments. Its use has actually been tape-recorded as far back as Egyptian times. Aloe has actually been made use of topically and also by mouth.

Its essences are usually used in cosmetics as well as can be located in whatever from fragrances to cream.

Aloe vera gel is located when you burst the leaves. It's commonly acknowledged as a natural remedy for minor scrapes as well as burns.

Some individuals think that juice from the aloe vera plant may have a similar calming impact for people with acid reflux. Aloe juices are discovered in the aloe latex. This is originated from the internal lining of the plant's fallen leaves.

Advantages Of Using Aloe Vera For Acid Reflux Symptoms

What are the advantages of utilizing aloe vera as a remedy for acid reflux?

Aloe vera is a tried and tested, all-natural acid reflux remedy that works in lowering GERD signs without any damaging events calling for withDr.awal.1 This may be a better choice for people than proton-pump preventions (PPIs) in particular situations. This is of terrific benefit with the expanding list of negative effects connected with long-lasting PPI usage.

- Aloe vera's antibacterial substances deal with poor germs in the gastrointestinal system to reduce the instance of SIBO, H. pylori, and also yeast. The gas created by poor bacteria can trigger bloating of the abdominal area as well as belching. Both weaken the LES closure to enable acid into the oesophagus, creating heartburn. Bad microorganisms also minimize the gastrointestinal system's ability to synthesize particular digestion enzymes, lowers the small intestine's capability to damage down healthy proteins into amino acids, as well as avoids nutrition absorption. Reductions in gastrointestinal function slow down the gastrointestinal process creating irregular bowel movements. Irregularity causes stomach pressure which in turn endangers the LES closure permitting tummy acid to leak through, reflux, right into the oesophagus.

- It boosts blood circulation, which aids boost the digestive system procedure.
- It supplies vital vitamins and amino acids that assist improve digestive functions.
- It's anti-inflammatory residential or commercial properties lower pain as well as calm the aggravated cellular lining of the oesophagus to ease heartburn.
- Its antibacterial substances promote the recovery of harmed or swollen cells.
- It also advertises recovery by boosting the immune system, minimizing inflammation, boosting circulation, and providing nutrients.

- It can be used as a laxative. Depending on your digestion demands, this might aid alleviate constipation and also stomach stress that results in indigestion. If you are not constipated, it's ideal to acquire a type that has the laxative component of the aloe plant removed.

Benefits of aloe vera juice

Pros

- Aloe vera has anti-inflammatory residential or commercial properties.
- The juice is filled with vitamins, minerals, and also amino acids.
- Aloe vera juice may increase digestion and also eliminate toxins from the body.
- Aloe vera has anti-inflammatory properties. This is why it's frequently utilized to treat sunburns or various other minor irritations.
- • Vitamins, minerals and amino acids are used to fill the water. Because of this, the juice is claimed to detox the body when taken inside. It may enhance food digestion as well as eliminate waste.

Aloe vera juice might also assist:

- lower cholesterol
- reduce blood sugar degrees
- promote hair growth
- invigorate skin

Finest Aloe Vera Forms For Acid Reflux

Use aloe vera created for inner usage just! Aloe vera for inner use can be acquired as supplements in a range of kinds: juice, gel, powder, and softgels.

Aloe vera gel, as well as juice, are best for heartburn therapy, though powder form may be mixed with water. These 3 forms have been available in direct call with the oesophagus assisting to decrease the inflammation of heartburn and also advertise healing of the oesophagal lining.

Aloe vera in soft gel and also pill form will certainly not deal with the oesophagus straight.

As pointed out in the above section, all these aloe vera kinds promote healing of the digestion system.

Aloe vera can be purchased with the laxative buildings removed. This is finest for a lot of instances as there are less adverse effects.

Exactly How To Use Aloe Vera For Acid Reflux

Aloe vera dosage will vary depending upon item supplier, the effectiveness of the item, as well as whether the laxative residential properties have actually been gotten rid of. Consult your pharmacist, product, and doctor label for directions on how to take your certain aloe vera supplement.

Aloe can be taken prior to dishes for avoidance or for therapy after heartburn has begun.

Softgels are likely to be taken numerous times a day with water. Sometimes they are taken prior to dishes to help with food digestion and heartburn prevention.

Aloe vera juice, gel, as well as a powder mixed with water might be taken prior to meals to aid with food digestion as well as heartburn prevention or after heartburn occurs as a remedy.

Revitalizing aloe vera beverages can also be made from aloe vera juice, powder, as well as gel. These three aloe vera forms can be combined with various other natural heartburn treatments like apple cider vinegar or with juices that will not advertise heartburn.

If you experience any adverse effects or pain of any kind of kind, discontinue use and consult your doctor. Your doctor might determine to alter your therapy routine. Know the threats and warnings of taking aloe vera internally

Just How To Make Aloe Vera Juice For Heartburn Relief

When making your very own Aloe vera juice be highly knowledgeable about the Warnings and threats detailed in the area over.

See to it you're growing the ideal aloe plant. You want to be making use of the Aloe vera species. There are other aloe plants that look similar to Aloe vera however they do not provide the exact same medicinal buildings.

You'll require to gather a large, healthy and balanced leaf. With a sharp blade, cut the leaf from the plant at its base.

LaunDr.y the fallen leave and area it levels side up on a reducing board.

With a sharp knife, trim the tough external layer with rind to expose the clear internal gel. You do not want the yellow-coloured skin. This layer has the latex, which is a strong laxative.

Scoop out the clear gel into a dish with a spoon and also aim to make sure you have actually not dug any one of the yellow-coloured peels.

To make aloe juice, combine 1-- 2 tablespoons of the aloe gel with 4-- 8 oz of water or coconut water. The amount of water will certainly rely on you. I like to have a higher level of Aloe vera when making use of the juice as a heartburn remedy as well as choose 4 ounces.

It can be stored in the refrigerator for up to a week if you want to make larger quantities.

Know its potential laxative impact. You should think about buying Aloe vera with the latex got rid of if you have problems due to the latex.

If you have adverse effects, terminate use immediately and also talk to your medical professional.

When Using Aloe Vera For Acid Reflux, threats And Warnings

Before using aloe vera as a remedy for acid reflux, talk to your medical professional. Usually, it is considered safe when using Aloe with latex (a part that has laxative properties), but it focuses closely on warnings and specific risks.

Aloe is not considered to be a risk-free long-term treatment for heartburn or various other internal disorders.

Aloe must not be taken in huge doses. Dosages of aloe with latex at 1 gram daily can be deadly. Huge does trigger kidney failure, heart problems, blood in the urine, diarrhoea, reduced potassium, muscle weakness, and weight management.

Mothers who are expectant or breastfeeding ought to not take aloe vera. Aloe can promote uterine contractions to trigger losing the unborn baby. It may additionally increase the threat of beginning fatality and skeletal abnormalities.

ChilDr.en and infants need to not be fed aloe items without doctor supervision.

Aloe vera can interfere with medicines, do not take without consulting with your doctor and also a pharmacist.

Do not take aloe if you are preparing to have a surgical procedure. It has been known to lower blood clotting.

Aloe ought to not be taken by diabetics. It may lower blood sugar level as well as can influence diabetic person Dr.ug.

Certain kinds of aloe vera can trigger diarrhoea. If you are taking various other diuretics or laxatives, prevent all aloe vera kinds with the latex part still undamaged.

Aloe can worsen problems such as piles, ulcerative colitis, Crohn's disease, or bowel blockage.

Do not take aloe if you dislike lily household plant team. It belongs to the lily family.

11. Rice

Dull starches are great options when it involves foods that are simple on the stomach cellular lining, according to SF Gate. Plain pasta, baked potatoes, as well as bread are various other good options too-- just be sure not to pack them up with butter or other acidic, high-fat condiments that might trigger heartburn.

12. Eco-friendly Vegetables

" Vegetables such as broccoli and also celery are low acidic foods," Warren states. "As an outcome, they can relieve the oesophagal lining." Other good veggies consist of asparagus and also environment-friendly beans,

Keeps in mind that typically, fresh, frozen, and canned veggies are risk-free for individuals with acid reflux. However, if those veggies are fried or creamed, the enhancement of high-fat components might aggravate the tummy.

13. Low-Acid Fruits

"While many fruits are acidic,adding to acid reflux, low-acid fruits are a great wager," Warren claims. Low-acid fruits consist of bananas and melons such as watermelon, cantaloupe, and honeydew.

Some fruits you might want to steer clear of are oranges, grapefruits, lemons, limes, tomatoes, and pineapples, Healthline says. These foods are very acidic and can trigger heartburn signs and symptoms.

Consuming such foods may help to prevent reflux of acid, however, to keep the signs and symptoms in check, ensure that various other foods like coffee, citrus, alcohol, chilled food and also spicy foods are prevented.

14. Apple cider vinegar

While there isn't enough study to prove that Dr.inking apple cider vinegar helps acid reflux, lots of people vouch that it helps. You must never Dr.ink it at full focus because it's a strong acid that can aggravate the oesophagus. Instead, placed a percentage in warm water as well as Dr.ink it with dishes.

15. Lemon water

Lemon juice is generally considered really acidic. However, a small amount of lemon juice blended with cosy water and honey has an alkalizing effect that reduces the effects of tummy acid. Likewise, honey has all-natural antioxidants, which safeguard the health and wellness of cells.

If you notice heartburn signs, it might be a good concept to change up your food options to ensure that you can really feel better and also a lot more comfortable after a scrumptious dish. Cochrane suggests consuming gradually, consuming smaller sized, much more regular meals throughout the day, as well as waiting at least three hours after consuming prior to lying down. Inevitably, if acid reflux is getting in the method of living your life, you must talk to your doctor regarding methods you can manage it.

" If you discover that any natural remedy needs to be utilized an increasing number of regularly to handle signs of reflux, it's time to speak with a physician about what you can do to far better take care of those symptoms," Cochrane says. "Uncontrolled reflux can trigger damages to the oesophagus and boost the danger of more health problems in time."

FOOD TO THE ACID REFLUX DIET

Among the most effective methods to heal your heartburn naturally is to stay clear of all the foods that create acid reflux.

There are several foods that might be accountable for your indigestion, as they trigger your belly to generate more acid to digest it.

You initially experience with heartburn isn't just agonizing, it's startling-- as well as perplexing. Especially when you realize that not only did last evening's glass of red wine set your reflux off, however, this morning's mimosa-and-avocado-toast breakfast left you downing Pepto, as well. Seriously, what provides?

Okay, as Felice Schnoll-Sussman, MD, a gastroenterologist at New York-Presbyterian Hospital, told us a few months ago, there are some simple things you can do at home to make your indigestion less persistent. To beginners, you're going to discover some basic standards that food can cause heartburn.

Belly acid is really coming up out of your stomach and also into your oesophagus when you have acid reflux. So you'll intend to avoid any kind of foods that are acidic or that cause your tummy to produce even more acid. That includes such tasty items as citrus fruit, fried chicken, and, ugh, white wine-- together with much more.

You do not always require to stop eating these completely (I mean, come on). However, if you've just recently taken care of a spell of reflux as well as you're looking for means to prevent extra, it's worth attempting to reduce on those foods or to reduce them out of your diet plan till you feel much better.

Nonetheless, not every person has the very same trigger foods, and not everyone is caused to the same degree. So it may take some trial-and-error prior to you figure out your own. And also absolutely do not be reluctant to bring in the assistance of your medical professional or a gastroenterologist on this quest. Ahead, see a couple of usual reflux-causing foods to aid you to suss out which ones require to go.

The checklist of acid response food to avoid that you will find below will help you to recognize which foods ought to be removed from your diet plan in order to handle your acid reflux normally:

Fatty Meat

Many fatty types of meat you will find in the supermarket will be on the acid reflux food checklist to stop.

The factor for this is that fat is extremely tough for your belly to digest, so it has to create even more acid in order to attempt to damage down the fatty bits. Wish to protect against heartburn? Change any kind of fatty meats with proteins that are low in fat.

Coffee

The largest issue with coffee is that the extra you Dr.ink, the even more acid you're revealing your digestive system to-- and it's not exactly very easy to stop at one mug. Not also decaf is secure for reflux patients.

The best approach for coffee enthusiasts is to stick to one mug, see just how it goes, and switch to tea if you need a little a lot more high levels of caffeine. Some patients still report concerns with tea. However,you've obtained a better fired with a mug of that than a latte.

Vegetables and also fruits-- That's right, there are fruits and vegetables that can be bad for you, yet only when you have heartburn. The reason that these foods are so negative for you is that they additionally create your tummy to create acid, as well as they themselves, have acids that include in your gastric acids in your belly. These include all citrus fruits and also juices, cranberry juice, tomatoes, French fried potatoes, salad, as well as raw onions.

Tomatoes

Tomato and also tomato-based items (e.g. pizza sauce) are on the naughty listing, too, because they're acidic. Tomatoes include 2 types of acid-- malic and also citric acid-- which can both cause reflux on their own.

Chocolate

There's more than one compound in delicious chocolate that adds to reflux. As Health discusses, we can blame the high levels of caffeine, theobromine, and also fat content in chocolate for this injustice. You could have better luck with delicious dark chocolate since it consists of less fat, but many individuals with reflux are stuck going without chocolate totally.

Fats and also Sweets

As stated over, fats are tough for the belly to absorb; as a result, more acid needs to be generated to manage fat usage. Desserts are also really tough on your tummy, and you would do well to stay clear of practically all type of sugary foods as well as fats.

Anything fried, deep-fried, containing great deals of butter, or very sweet are all on the no-no listing.

High-fat foods of any kind are no-nos when you're dealing with reflux. It involves meats, cheeses and anything fried. Yet, believe it, or otherwise, the avocados and nuts fall into this mulch as well. (This is one time when it does not truly matter whether your fats are "healthy" or not.) So when the next burger-and-guac evening appears, you're likely to have to do a cost-benefit evaluation on whether it's actually worth it.

Alcohol

The study is surprisingly split when it concerns alcohol. Some research studies suggest that there's no organization in between moderate alcohol consumption and also reflux, while others reveal that some kinds of alcohol (white wine and hard liquor specifically) are even worse wrongdoers than others.

So we would certainly recommend trying to remove alcohol if you have a reflux flareup, yet don't necessarily expect to do so to be a magic bullet.

Strong Dr.ink

Yes, like Samson in the Bible, you should avoid strong Dr.ink if you have indigestion.

The explanation for this is that strong beverages such as coffee, tea, soda, and power Dr.inks all consist of a lot of sugar; however, they are also highly acidic, as well as include in the acid content of your stomach.

Peppermint

If you have a dismaying stomach many thanks to indigestion, peppermint may assist calm it down since it can alleviate your stomach muscles and the flow of bile. If you're dealing with reflux particularly, you should avoid the mint-- those same leisure results likewise act on the sphincter in between your oesophagus and also tummy, making it much easier for acid to slip its means up.

Dairy products

Most full-fat milk items, in fact, have an extremely high-fat material, as well as some of them even have a great deal of sugar. While dairy consists of great deals of essential nutrients, the fat is not very crucial.

You need to remove all full-fat dairy from your diet regimen, especially ice cream, sour lotion, whole milk, cream cheese, and home cheese.

Late-night snacks

 Avoid consuming anything in both hours prior to you go to bed. Likewise, you can try eating four to 5 smaller sized dishes throughout the day rather than a couple of big meals.

Garlic And Onions

These 2 veggies are terrific for including an added delicious kick to your favourite meals, yet they can additionally increase your reflux. Raw onions are especially infamous for boosting the level of acidity in your oesophagus, so prepare those babies if you can.

Grains

Refined grains are really hard on your tummy, and also they are known to add to heartburn.

You need to specifically stay clear of white flour, in addition to a lot of the items made with polished flour.

Others:

- Citrus fruits
- Refined sugar
- Spicy food
- Caffeine
- spearmint
- Carbonated Dr.inks, like soda

Gluten (study suggests that a gluten-free diet can assist resolve acid reflux signs and symptoms)

Other suggestions that could assist include consuming a number of smaller dishes a day instead of 1-2 big meals and not eating near bedtime, so your body has time to absorb before lying down.

Yes, I know this listing of food has a lot of your favoured things, but the good news is that by doing so you can prevent your GERD from getting worse.

LESS THAN 30 DAY TREATMENT AND RECIPES FOR ACID REFLUX

Your diet for heartburn is just one of the most crucial things that you can do to avoid indigestion from getting out of control or being as well unpleasant.

Bear in mind that it is the food you consume that is triggering the manufacturing of acid in your belly, and also, therefore, it is your duty to put the ideal foods in your mouth.

You already understand what foods you need to eliminate your diet plan, yet here are some foods that you must contribute to your diet regimen for acid reflux:

Fibre

Fibre is just one of the most vital things to contribute to your heartburn treatment.

Nutritional fibre assists in taking in the acid in your belly and will send it on its means down the intestinal tracts.Make sure you get nutrients from fruit, vegetables, and whole grains that will not aggravate your heartburn or acid reflux, as well as try to prevent food items that contain large amounts of starch and also sugar.

Protein

Did you recognize that foods that are abundant in healthy protein will assist in strengthening the muscular tissues of your stomach and oesophagus to stop the acid from coming back up?

It is important to prevent healthy eating proteins that are really high in fat, so you must try to find low-fat protein sources like fish, egg whites, skinless hen or turkey, legumes, and also really low-fat meats in your indigestion therapy.

Pineapple

While pineapple should be taken into consideration one of the most acidic fruits on earth, it is, in fact, excellent for your heartburn.

The factor for this is that it contains bromelain, which is superb to help your food digestion, lower your acid response, and also calm your stomach down.

Papaya

This exotic fruit is highly recommended by physicians, as it consists of papain.

This enzyme located in papayas improves your digestion as well as assists to manage the absorption of protein in your body. It can help to lower your indigestion, enhance your digestion, and bring peace to your tummy.

These are just a few of one of the most important foods, but you would do well to go further and also enhance your diet regimen considerably.

Much less than 30 days Meal Plan and Tips to Stop Heartburn

There's even more to dissuading the pain than staying clear of particular foods and Dr.inks if you're one of the 15 million Americans experiencing heartburn every day.

Heartburn relief also relates to the timing as well as the size of your meals, claims The American College of Gastroenterology, which is why planning your dishes can be so essential. Yet before we get to the preparation part, it aids to recognize what creates heartburn.

Dish Planning Tips Preventing Heartburn

If you have frequent or occasional heartburn, you can help reduce the propensity of the LES to kick back, and decrease the possibility that the belly materials (and also the belly acid) will surely spray towards the LES by remembering a few points:

- Avoid lying down for two to three hrs after consuming. When you lie down, it's literally simpler for stomach materials to sprinkle up toward the LES. By staying up or standing, gravity aids tolerate materials stay where they belong-- at the end of the tummy.
- Avoid products that deteriorate the LES muscular tissue (like delicious chocolate, peppermint, caffeine, alcohol, fatty foods) as well as foods and Dr.inks that may irritate a damaged oesophagus cellular lining (citrus and also citrus juice, tomatoes as well as tomato juice, and also chilli peppers as well as black pepper).
- Avoid eating large meals since the extra quantity in the stomach, the most likely the stomach contents will certainly sprinkle toward the LES. Try eating four to 5 small meals as opposed to 2 or 3 huge ones.
- Because they have a tendency to remain in the tummy much longer; fried or greasy foods can

also weaken the LES muscle, avoid high-fat meals.

- Stay clear of cigarette smoking and also prevent alcohol before, throughout, or after meals that seem to lead to heartburn (like dinner). Both smoking cigarettes and also alcohol deteriorate the LES muscle mass.
- Try waiting at least 2 hours after a dish prior to exercising if you locate your heartburn seems to get worse after exercise.
- Chew periodontal (a non-peppermint taste) after dishes to promote saliva manufacturing (the bicarbonate in saliva counteracts acid) and also enhance peristalsis (which assists relocate the tummy materials right into the little intestine faster).
- Plan your meals to urge certain however sluggish fat burning if you are obese. Extra weight around the stomach, specifically, can push against the belly and also boost the stress increasing toward the LES.
- Consume alcohol a little glass of water at the end of dishes to help dilute and also clean down any kind of belly acid that could be splashing up into the oesophagus, suggests Shekhar Challa, MD, head of state of Kansas Medical Clinic as well as writer of Spurn The Burn: Treat The Heat.

Intend on heartburn-friendly Dr.inks like water, mineral water, decaffeinated tea, noncitrus juices, or nonfat or low-fat milk. Dr.inks to avoid consist of:

Soft Dr.inks: These can bloat the abdomen, enhancing the stress in the stomach and also motivating stomach acid to splash up right into the oesophagus.

Juices: Tomato and also citrus juices can aggravate a damaged oesophagus.

Alcohols, coffee (also decaf) as well as caffeinated tea and soda pop can enhance the acid web content in the belly as well as relax the LES.

Eat a high fibre diet plan! A current study located that individuals that complied with a high-fibre dish plan were 20% less likely to have acid reflux symptoms, no matter their body weight. You'll discover fibre in whole grains, fruits, vegetables, beans, seeds as well as nuts (basically unprocessed plant foods).

27 DAYS GASTRIC REFLUX DIET RECIPES

BREAKFASTS

Dairy-Free Pancake

Ingredients

- 1 cup of versatile flour
- 2 teaspoons baking powder
- 1 cup unsweetened almond milk
- 1 large egg
- 1 large egg yolk
- 1 1/2 teaspoons canola oil
- 2 tablespoons sugar
- 1 can spray cooking oil

Instructions

- Include damp ingredients and Dr.y active ingredients alternately. Keep mixing until all contents are included
- Spray pan with oil then pour the mix
- Cook until soft brown or no bubbles are revealing

Omelette

Ingredients

- 2 big eggs
- Minced mushrooms (or any other alkaline vegetable)
- Diced spinach (or any other leafy green).
- Salt and pepper to taste

Instructions

- Whisk both eggs into a bowl, then add veggies. You might also select to brown the veggies for 5 minutes before including them to the egg mixture
- Heat oil in a pan
- Pour mix and wait on the omelette to form

No-Bake Faux Banana Bread

Components

- 4 large ripe bananas
- 1 large egg
- 2 tsp honey (optional)
- 1 can spray oil
- 1 tbsp cinnamon powder

Guidelines

- Mash ripe bananas onto a bowl, then include egg. Whisk together. Add cinnamon powder and honey.
- Spray pan with oil.
- Put mix onto the pan and await it to form.

Tater Tots

Active ingredients

- 1/4 cup carrots
- 1/4 cup sweet potato
- 1/4 squash
- 1 tablespoon flour
- Salt and pepper to taste

Directions

- Preheat oven to 450 degrees Fahrenheit
- Peel and boil carrots, sweet potato, and squash. When soft, Dr.ain, and shred
- Mix veggies with pepper, salt, and flour
- Form into little balls and bake for 20 minutes or till golden brown

Fabulous French Toast

Components

- 3 eggs
- 1 cup low-fat milk
- 1 teaspoon vanilla extract
- 1/2 teaspoon cinnamon
- Pinch of salt
- 8 pieces 100 per cent whole-grain bread, heavily sliced
- 1 cup low-fat, plain yoghurt
- 1 banana, sliced
- 1 tablespoon pure maple syrup

Direction

- In a large blending bowl, including the eggs, milk, vanilla, cinnamon, and salt. Whisk till smooth.
- Heat a cast-iron frying pan over medium heat.
- Soak the bread pieces in the egg mixture till saturated, about 30 seconds each side.
- Prepare in batches till the bread turns golden brown, about 4 minutes each side. Repeat until all the pieces are cooked.
- Top the French toast with dollops of yoghurt and bananas. Dr.izzle the maple syrup on top.
- Per serving: Calories 322 (From Fat 66); Fat 7g (Saturated 3g); Cholesterol 146mg; Sodium

475mg; CarbohyDr.ate 49g (Dietary Fiber 5g); Protein 17g.

Pear Banana Nut Muffins

Active ingredients

- 1 medium pear, peeled and diced
- 2 tablespoons pear nectar
- 1 cup whole-wheat flour
- 1 cup rolled oats
- 1 tablespoon ground flaxseed
- 3 tablespoons maple sugar flakes or Sucanat (optional)
- 1 teaspoon baking powder
- 1/2 teaspoon baking soda
- 1 teaspoon cinnamon
- 1/4 teaspoon cardamom.
- 1/4 teaspoon sea salt
- 2 eggs
- 1/3 cup vanilla almond milk
- 2 tablespoons butter, melted
- 2 teaspoons vanilla
- 1 medium banana, peeled and mashed
- 1 cup sliced walnuts

Instructions

- Preheat the oven to 375 degrees F. Line a 12-cup muffin pan with paper liners or grease the pan with olive oil; reserved.
- Lower the heat to low and simmer for 3 minutes. Let the mixture cool for 15 minutes.
- In a big bowl, combine the flour, oats, flaxseed, sugar flakes (if wanted), baking powder, baking soda, cinnamon, cardamom, and sea salt. Mix well.
- In a small bowl, combine the cooled pear mix, eggs, almond milk, banana, vanilla, and butter; mix well.
- Add the pear mixture to the Dr.y active ingredients and stir simply up until integrated. Stir in the walnuts. Spoon the batter into the ready muffin pan.
- Bake for 15 to 20 minutes, or up until the muffins are set and gently browned. Eliminate the muffins from the pan and cool them on a cake rack.
- Per serving: Calories 180 (From Fat 92); Fat 10g (Saturated 2g); Cholesterol 41mg; Sodium 185mg; CarbohyDr.ate 18g; Dietary Fiber 3g; Protein 5g.

Skillet Peanut Butter Cinnamon Spice Cookie

Ingredients

- 1 big egg
- 1 cup natural peanut butter
- 1/2 cup brown sugar
- 1/4 cup almond meal
- 1 teaspoon vanilla extract
- 1 teaspoon baking soda
- 1 teaspoon cinnamon
- 1/4 teaspoon ground ginger
- 1/4 teaspoon salt
- Non-stick spray
- 2 tablespoons peanuts, optional, for garnish

Preparation

Preheat oven to 350 F

- In a big bowl, beat egg up until a little frothy. Whisk in the peanut butter, brown sugar, almond meal, vanilla extract, baking soda, cinnamon, ginger, and salt until well integrated.
- Spray an ovenproof skillet gently with nonstick spray. Put batter into the skillet and spread evenly with a spatula. Spray the leading with a few peanuts and press down somewhat if wanted.
- Place cookie on a rack embedded in the centre of the oven and bake 10-12 minutes up until

puffed and golden around the edges. Let cool 10 minutes before cutting and serving.

Basic Vegetable and Chicken Wonton Soup

Components

- 2 tablespoons olive oil
- 1 small onion, combined or finely minced
- 1 tablespoon newly grated ginger
- 1 clove garlic, grated
- 1 pound ground chicken
- 1/4 teaspoon salt
- 48 square wonton wrappers
- 10 cups water
- 3/4 teaspoon kosher salt
- 1/4 teaspoon ground black pepper
- 1 tablespoon red wine vinegar
- 1/2 teaspoon red pepper flakes
- 16 medium cremini mushroom caps, sliced
- 4 small carrots, sliced into rounds
- 1 cup frozen, shelled edamame
- 5 scallions, sliced (optional)

Preparation

- Heat a medium pan over medium-high heat. Heat oil till shiny and swirl to coat the pan. Sauté the onion, ginger, and garlic for about 4 minutes. Transfer to a big bowl.

- Include ground chicken and salt to the onion mix. Stir well (utilize your hands!).
- Set out a brush, shallow dish with water, and a lined baking sheet at your workstation. Working with one wonton at a time, spoon 1/2 tablespoon of the chicken mixture into the centre of the wonton wrapper. Brush the sides with water and fold into a triangle, pointer pointing away from you.
- Integrate water, salt, pepper, red wine vinegar, and red pepper flakes in a big pot. Give a boil, then lower heat to a simmer.
- Add mushrooms, carrots, edamame, and dumplings. Give a simmer and let cook for 20 minutes. Serve sprayed with sliced up scallions, if preferred.

Breaded and Baked Homemade Chicken Nuggets

Active ingredients

- 1 pound boneless, skinless chicken breast, cut into 1x2-inch rectangles
- 1 large egg

* 1/2 teaspoon garlic powder
* 1/2 teaspoon kosher salt
* 1/2 cup plain breadcrumbs
* 1 1/4 cups riced cauliflower

Preparation

* Preheat oven to 350F. Line a large baking tray and set aside until prepared to use.
* In a little shallow plate, integrate egg, garlic powder, and salt. Blend well to integrate.
* In a separate plate, integrate breadcrumbs and cauliflower.
* Dip the chicken pieces into the egg mixture. If required), let the excess Dr.ip off prior to the finish with the breadcrumb and cauliflower mix (you can pat it on to assist it in sticking. Set up the layered pieces on the ready flat pan.
* Bake for 20 minutes, turning as soon as midway through.

Roasted Root Veggie Breakfast Tacos

Components

* 1 small sweet potatoes, cubed (1/4" - 1/2" pieces).

- 1 medium carrot, peeled and sliced (1/4" rounds).
- 1 tablespoon olive oil.
- 1 teaspoon ground cumin.
- 1/2 teaspoon ground coriander.
- 1/4 teaspoon salt.
- Zest of 1/2 lime.
- 1 cup canned black beans (mashed).
- 2 (6-inch) corn tortillas.

Preparation

- Preheat oven to 350 F and line a little baking sheet with parchment paper.
- In a little bowl, mix the sweet potatoes and carrots with olive oil, cumin, salt, coriander, and lime zest. Transfer to the baking sheet and roast for 15 minutes.
- Once the vegetables are ready, spread the mashed black beans on the tortilla and top with the veggies.
- See the serving ideas below for additional topping recommendations.

Serving Tips

The roasted vegetables take off with taste, so you can easily delight in these breakfast tacos without anything included. They'll feel more like breakfast topped with an egg or lime-zested yoghurt. You can include a fried egg, cooked in half a teaspoon of olive oil, and sprinkle with a little bit of lime passion for an additional 90 calories. Top with 2 tablespoons plain low-fat yoghurt blended with zest from half a lime for an extra 35 calorie.

Strawberry Basil Sparkler

Active ingredients

- Ice
- 4 strawberries, sliced
- 6 basil leaves, approximately chopped
- 12 ounces sodium-free carbonated water

Preparation

- Add ice to a highball glass
- Add chopped strawberries and basil
- Fill with sparkling water and stir

Component Variations and Substitutions

Use any kind of fruit or herbs that you like, such as blueberries, blackberries, citrus fruit, or apples, with mint or thyme. You can chew on them after, so pick your favourite!

You can likewise utilize plain water if you 'd rather.

Cooking and Serving Tips

Ensure your carbonated water is unflavored and sodium complimentary so that your last Dr.ink is nutrition-friendly.

Chia Pudding With Honeydew Melon

Components

- 1 cup of vanilla soy milk
- 1/4 cup chia seeds
- 1/2 cup finely sliced honeydew melon

Preparation

- Combine soy milk and chia seeds in a bowl and blend well.
- Cover with plastic wrap and transfer to the refrigerator. Allow setting for 2 hours.

- After 2 hours, mix carefully and return to the fridge to chill for 2 more hours, or up to overnight.
- Melon lead before serving.

Roasted Veggie and Goat Cheese Frittata

Ingredients

- 1/2 medium zucchini, diced in medium pieces
- 1/2 cup small broccoli florets
- 1 medium carrot, diced in small pieces
- 1/2 small sweet potato, diced in small pieces
- 1/2 cup baby Bella mushrooms, sliced
- 1 teaspoon basil
- 1/2 teaspoon thyme
- 1 teaspoon oregano
- 1/4 teaspoon salt
- 1 tablespoon olive oil
- 4 large eggs
- 1/8 teaspoon turmeric
- 1/4 cup goat cheese, crumbled

Preparation

- Preheat oven to 350F
- Add all of the chopped veggies to a greased 9-inch cake pan and toss with basil, thyme, oregano, salt, and olive oil. Roast for about 15 to 20 minutes, up until the sweet potato and carrots are softened.

- In a small bowl whisk together eggs, turmeric, and fell apart goat cheese.
- Get rid of the vegetables from the oven and utilize a spoon to distribute them throughout the pan uniformly.
- Put the egg mixture over the vegetables and cook for another 5 to 10 minutes, up until the eggs are set.
- Eliminate from oven and let cool. Slice and serve!

Sweet Potato Toast With Ginger-Honey Almond Butter and Kiwi

Ingredients

- 1 medium sweet potato, peeled or unpeeled
- 3 tablespoons almond butter
- 1/2 teaspoon honey
- 1/4 teaspoon ground ginger
- 2 medium kiwi, peeled or unpeeled

Preparation

- Slice sweet potato-lengthwise into 1/4-inch slices.
- In a little bowl, stir almond ginger, honey, and butter together up until combined.

- Toast sweet potato pieces on the toaster's high setting till the sweet potato slices are soft and cooked through. Note, you may need to toast 2 or more times to get them to this state.
- Spread one side of each piece of the roasted sweet potato slices with the almond-ginger-honey mixture and top with kiwi slices.

Papaya Yogurt & Walnut Boat

Ingredients

- 1 medium papaya, halved
- 1/2 cup plain fat-free or low-fat Greek yoghurt
- 1/4 cup walnuts
- 1/4 teaspoon ground cinnamon

Preparation

- Scoop out the seeds of the papaya.
- Fill each papaya half with half of the yoghurt, walnut halves, and dust with ground cinnamon.
- Eat with a spoon, scooping out bites of papaya flesh.

Oven-Dr.ied Persimmon Rounds

Ingredients

6 medium Fuyu persimmons

Preparation

- Preheat oven to 250F.
- Very finely slice the persimmons crosswise into 1/4-inch rounds.
- Divide the persimmons between 2 cake rack set atop baking sheets.
- Bake till the centres look Dr.y, and the edges begin to huddle about 1 1/2 to 2 hours.
- Store in an airtight container in the refrigerator.

Cran-Apple Carrot Muffins

Ingredients

- 1.25 cups entire wheat flour
- 1/2 cup brown sugar
- 1/2 teaspoon baking powder
- 1/2 teaspoon baking soda
- 1 teaspoon cinnamon

- 1/2 teaspoon salt
- 1 cup rolled oats
- 1 tablespoon ground flaxseed
- 2.5 tablespoons water
- 3 tablespoons olive oil
- 1/3 cup non-fat plain Greek yoghurt
- 1/2 cup applesauce
- 4 medium carrots, grated (about 1 3/4 to 2 cups worth).
- 1/2 cup fresh cranberries, approximately sliced.

Preparation

- Preheat oven to 400F. Spray a 12-cup muffin tin with cooking spray and reserved.
- Whisk together the flour, sugar, baking powder, baking soda, cinnamon and salt. Stir in the oats.
- In a little bowl, mix together the ground flaxseed with water. Let sit for a minimum of 5 minutes for it to begin to gel.
- Add the olive oil, yoghurt, and applesauce to the "flax egg" and blend together. Discard into the Dr.y ingredients together with the cranberries and carrots.
- Utilizing a rubber spatula, stir till the mix is simply combined. Do not over-mix otherwise, and the muffins will come out tough.
- Spoon the batter evenly among the muffin tin and bake for 24 to 28 minutes, till the tops are

puffed and golden, and a toothpick inserted in the centre comes out tidy. Let cool on a cake rack.

Mixed Berry Ice Cubes With Seltzer

Ingredients

- 1/4 cup blueberries
- 1/4 cup raspberries
- 1/4 cup blackberries
- tap water
- sparkling water

Preparation

- Divide the berries amongst a 16 cube ice cube tray. Include tap water to cover and place in the freezer till frozen (best to do this a day ahead).
- Put the appropriate quantity of ice cubes in a glass and top with seltzer.

Do It Yourself Bagels: A Simple 6-Ingredient Recipe

Ingredients

- 1 1/2 cups warm water

- 1 package Dr.y active yeast
- 1 tablespoon granulated sugar
- 3 1/2 cups bread flour
- 2 teaspoons kosher salt
- 1 egg

Preparation

- In a medium bowl whisk warm water, yeast, and sugar; reserved for 10 minutes.
- In the bowl of an electric mixer fitted with a dough hook, combine flour and salt.
- Include yeast mix to the flour and mix on medium speed for 6 to 8 minutes, till the dough is formed into a large, smooth ball.
- Move dough to an oiled bowl (coconut oil is working well).
- Cover with a clean dish towel and allow to increase for about one hour.
- Bring a big pot of water to a boil, preheat oven to 425F, and line 2 sheet pans with parchment paper.
- Transfer dough to a lightly floured surface and divide into 8 equal-sized pieces. Roll each piece of dough into a ball and utilizing fingers poke a hole in each piece; reserved and repeat with remaining pieces of dough.
- Reduce heat to a simmer when water is boiling.

- Operating in batches, place 3 bagels in the water and cook for one minute per side. Remove the bagel from the water using a slotted spoon and place into a prepared sheet pan.
- Integrate egg and one tablespoon of water in a small bowl and blend well. As soon as all bagels have actually been boiled, brush with egg wash.
- Bake bagels for 15 to 18 minutes or till golden brown
- Allow cooling for at least 10 minutes prior to serving.

Simple Grilled Vegetable Oreganata

Ingredients

- 1 tablespoon olive oil
- 1/2 teaspoon kosher salt
- 1 tablespoon of rice vinegar
- 2 tablespoons chopped fresh oregano
- 1 medium eggplant, peeled and sliced lengthwise
- 1 bell pepper, seeds and ribs eliminated, cut into big pieces
- 1 bunch asparagus, ends trimmed
- 1 large zucchini, chopped lengthwise

Preparation

- In a big bowl whisk olive oil, salt, vinegar, and sliced oregano.
- Location all vegetables into the bowl with marinade and toss to coat
- The heat outside grill or grill pan to medium-high.
- Location veggies on the grill.
- Prepare zucchini, eggplant, and pepper pieces for about 4 minutes per side.
- Toss asparagus gently on the grill and cook until tender. This will take 3 to 4 minutes as well.
- Transfer prepared veggies onto a large platter.
- Serve warm or at space temperature level.

Apple Crisp Dessert Recipe

Ingredients

- 4 medium apples (peeled, seeded, and diced)
- 1 teaspoon cornstarch
- 1 teaspoon cinnamon
- 1/2 lemon, juiced
- 1/4 teaspoon lemon passion (freshly grated)
- 2 tablespoons sugar
- 3 tablespoons saltless butter (cold, diced into small pieces)
- 2 tablespoons all-purpose flour
- 1.2 cup rolled oats
- 2 tablespoons light brown sugar (packed)

- 1/2 teaspoon kosher salt
- 1/3 cup sliced walnuts
- 6 tablespoons 100% apple juice

Preparation

- Preheat oven to 350F
- Spray 6 (5-ounce) ramekins with cooking spray and place on a baking sheet lined with parchment paper.
- In a medium bowl, integrate apples, cornstarch, cinnamon, lemon juice, lemon enthusiasm, and sugar.
- Toss well and set aside for 10 minutes.
- In a different bowl, combine butter, flour, oats, brown sugar, salt, and walnuts; mix well to integrate.
- Spoon apple mixture uniformly into ready ramekins, then sprinkle with topping.
- Lead every serving with an apple juice tablespoon.
- Place in the oven and bake for about 30 minutes or until golden and bubbly.
- Remove from the oven and enable to cool slightly before serving.

Buttermilk Ranch Dr.essing

Ingredients

- 1/2 cup low-fat buttermilk
- 1/4 cup mayonnaise
- 1/4 cup non-fat Greek yoghurt
- 2 tablespoons chopped fresh chives
- 2 tablespoons chopped fresh parsley
- 2 tablespoons freshly squeezed lemon juice
- 1 teaspoon fresh lemon zest
- 1 teaspoon garlic powder
- 1 teaspoon kosher salt
- 1/2 teaspoon black pepper

Preparation

- Combine buttermilk, mayo, and Greek yoghurt in a medium bowl or large glass measuring cup.
- Add chopped chives and parsley, followed by lemon juice and lemon enthusiasm, garlic powder, kosher salt, and black pepper.
- Whisk very well and place in the fridge to chill for a minimum of 20 minutes before serving.
- The Dr.essing can be stored in the fridge for as much as 1 week.

Lower Fat Pesto and Butternut Squash Pizza

Ingredients

- 1 bundle Dr.y active yeast
- 1 teaspoon sugar
- 1 cup of warm water
- 1 1/2 cups whole wheat pastry flour
- 1 1/2 cups all-purpose flour
- 1 teaspoon kosher salt
- 2 tablespoons additional virgin olive oil, divided
- 1 cup butternut squash, diced
- 1/2 tablespoon olive oil
- 1/4 teaspoon salt
- 3 tablespoons ready pesto (usage this dish for simple nut-free leafy green pesto)
- 1/2 cup part-skim mozzarella cheese, shredded
- 2 tablespoons Parmesan cheese, grated

Preparation

- Integrate yeast, sugar, and water in a small bowl or determining cup; permit and stir to sit for 10 minutes.

- To prepare the dough, place flours and salt in the bowl of an electric mixer fitted with a dough hook.
- Include the yeast mixture and one tablespoon of olive oil. Run maker on low until ingredients are simply combined, then increase speed medium for 6 to 8 minutes, till the dough has come together in a big ball.
- Transfer dough to an oiled bowl (using the very first tablespoon) and cover with a tidy cooking area towel. Let increase for one hour. Shop half the dough in a freezer-safe bag doe use another time.
- About midway through the dough rising, preheat oven to 400F and prepare a sheet pan lined with parchment paper.
- Place butternut squash on sheet pan and Dr.izzle with oil and spray with salt. Roast in the 400-degree oven until tender.
- If you have not already, prepare pesto at this time.
- Place raised dough on a lightly floured surface area and roll flat using a rolling pin. Thoroughly eliminate sheet pan from oven and Dr.izzle with olive oil (the second tablespoon).
- Transfer dough to pan and carefully press dough to the edges of the pan. Leading with pesto, prepared squash, and sprinkle with cheese.
- Raise the oven temperature level to 450F.

- Bake for 16 minutes, turning pan once half method through cooking.
- When cheese is bubbly, and crust is golden brown remove from oven and enables to cool slightly before slicing into 8 big pieces.

Crispy Baked French Fries

Ingredients

- 4 medium russet potatoes
- 1 tablespoon olive oil
- 1/2 teaspoon kosher salt
- 1/4 teaspoon freshly ground black pepper

Preparation

- Preheat oven to 400F.
- Line a baking sheet with parchment paper and reserve.
- Scrub potatoes well to remove any dirt, leaving the skins on.
- Slice longways into large slices.
- Cut again into uniformly sized sticks.
- Transfer to the ready baking sheet.
- Drizzle with olive oil and season with salt and pepper
- Toss well to disperse the spices.

- Bake for 35 to 40 minutes, tossing once or two times throughout cooking.
- When golden and crisp, remove from the oven and permit to cool somewhat before serving.

Whole Grain Wild Blueberry Muffins

Ingredients

- 1 1/2 cups + 2 tablespoons white entire wheat flour, divided
- 1/2 cup sugar
- 1/2 tablespoon baking powder (low salt if possible)
- 1 tablespoon lemon enthusiasm
- 1 cup unsweetened almond milk or skim milk
- 1/4 cup plain nonfat Greek yoghurt
- 2 large eggs
- 2 teaspoons vanilla extract
- 1 cup frozen wild blueberries

Preparation

- Heat oven to 400F. Spray a standard muffin tin with cooking spray or line with muffin liners, then spray with cooking spray.
- In a large bowl, whisk 1 1/2 cups flour, sugar, baking powder, and lemon passion.

- In a different bowl, whisk together wet ingredients. Put into Dr.y active ingredients and stir carefully up until just integrated.
- In a small bowl, toss blueberries with staying 2 tablespoons flour. Gently fold into the batter.
- Scoop batter into muffin tin, filling about 3/4 of the method full. Bake 15 to 20 minutes or until a toothpick inserted into the centre comes out clean.
- Cool 10 minutes before eliminating muffins from the pan

Overnight Oatmeal Recipe

Ingredients

- 1/2 cup skim milk or vanilla almond milk
- 1/4 cup plain nonfat Greek yoghurt
- 1 teaspoon honey
- 1 teaspoon vanilla
- 1/2 cup rolled oats
- 1/2 cup any fruit

Preparation

- In a container or another container with a cover, blend together milk, vanilla, honey, and yoghurt. Stir in oats. Cover and cool overnight or a minimum of 6 hours.
- In the early morning, stir in your preferred fruit and enjoy.

Strawberry Green Tea Ice Cubes

Ingredients

- 3 green tea bags
- 2 cups of water
- 1 tablespoon honey
- 1 cup thinly sliced strawberries

Preparation

- Heat water and brew tea.
- Mix in honey while still hot and stir to combine.
- Permit to cool at room temperature for one hour or place in the fridge (with the tea bags in the mixture) for up to 24 hours.
- Pour cooled tea mix into ice cube tray.
- Place ice cube tray in the freezer and allow to freeze for 15 minutes.

- As soon as 15 minutes have passed, and the cubes have begun to freeze, carefully include a few sliced strawberries to each cube.
- Return the tray to the freezer to freeze totally, about 3 hours.
- Once frozen, leave ice cubes in trays until prepared to transfer or use to a freezer-safe bag.

Low-Fat Peanut Butter and Banana Shake

Ingredients

- 1 medium banana, frozen and chopped
- 1 cup of coconut water
- 4 ounces plain nonfat Greek yoghurt
- 2 tablespoons powdered peanut butter

Preparation

- Place banana, coconut water, Greek yoghurt, and powdered peanut butter in a blender.
- Mix up until smooth.
- Serve instantly.

Overnight Oats With Bananas and Honey

Ingredients

- 1/2 cup rolled oats
- 1/2 cup unsweetened almond milk
- 1 teaspoon ground flaxseed
- 1 teaspoon honey
- 1/2 banana, sliced

Preparation

- In a little container, integrate oats, almond milk, flaxseed, and honey.
- Stir well to integrate.
- Cover container with a cover or plastic wrap and place in the refrigerator overnight
- Before serving, leading with banana and spray with more flax, if wanted.

Sweet and Crunchy Fennel and Apple Salad

Ingredients

- 1 bulb fennel, thinly sliced
- 1 sweet apple (like red scrumptious), unpeeled and thinly sliced
- 2 tablespoons additional virgin olive oil
- 2 teaspoons rice vinegar
- 1/4 teaspoon kosher salt

Preparation

- Put the fennel, apple, olive oil, and vinegar in a medium bowl.
- Season the active ingredients with salt, then toss carefully to combine.
- Serve chilled or at room temperature.

Cheesy Cauliflower Cakes

Ingredients

- 2 cups cauliflower (prepared)
- 1 egg (beaten)
- 1/2 cup Parmesan cheese (grated)
- 1 cup panko breadcrumbs

Preparation

- Preheat oven to 375 F.
- Line a baking sheet with parchment paper.
- In a big bowl combine cauliflower, egg, cheese, and breadcrumbs.
- Mash active ingredients with a fork until well mixed.
- Utilizing clean hands form into 8 cakes.
- Place cakes on a prepared baking sheet and spray the tops with cooking spray cooking.
- Bake for 20 minutes up until golden.

- Allow cooling somewhat before serving.

Light and Fluffy Angel Food Cupcakes

Ingredients

- 1/2 cup cake flour
- 1/4 cup powdered sugar
- 1/4 teaspoon kosher salt
- 6 big egg whites (room temperature)
- 1/2 teaspoon cream of tartar
- 1 teaspoon vanilla extract
- 1/2 cup granulated sugar

Preparation

- Preheat oven to 350F.
- Line a cupcake pan with paper liners; reserved.
- In a medium bowl sift cake flour, powdered sugar, and salt.
- Location egg whites in a different bowl and beat with an electrical mixture up until they begin to thicken.
- Include cream of tartar and vanilla and beat for about 2 minutes more or up until stiff peaks begin to form.
- Gradually gather sugar and continue to beat on high until all the sugar is included. Turn off

mixer and gently fold the flour mixture into egg whites using a rubber spatula.

- As soon as well mixed, spoon uniformly into cupcake pan.
- Bake for 12 to 15 minutes or until tops are gently golden and a toothpick from the centre of the cupcakes comes out clean.
- Put on a cake rack to cool completely.

Banana Ginger Energy Smoothie

Ingredients

- 1/2 cup ice
- 2 cups of milk
- 2 bananas, ripe
- 1 cup yoghurt
- 1/2 tsp. fresh ginger, peeled and grated fine
- 2 tablespoon.brown sugar or honey (optional)

Preparation

- In a mixer, add the ice, milk, yoghurt, bananas, and ginger.
- Mix up until smooth.
- Add sugar as required.

Gala Apple Honeydew Smoothie

Ingredients

- 2 cups honeydew melon (peeled, seeded, cut into chunks)
- 4 tbsp. fresh aloe vera, skin eliminated
- 1 Gala apple (peeled, cored, halved)
- 1/16 tsp. lime zest (use a grater to get the passion)
- 1 1/2 cups ice
- 1/4 tsp. salt

Preparation

- In a mixer, add the melon, ice, aloe vera, lime, apple, and salt passion.
- Start mixing on Pulse prior to switching to High. Stop and stir the mixture as needed to get a smooth consistency.

Muesli-Style Oatmeal

Ingredients

- 1 cup immediate oatmeal
- 1 cup of milk
- 2 tablespoon.raisins (given a boil, Dr.ained)
- 1/2 banana, diced
- 1/2 golden apple, peeled, diced
- Pinch of salt
- 2 tsp. sugar or honey

Preparation

- The evening before (or a minimum of 2 hours prior to), mix the oatmeal, milk, raisins, salt, and sugar (or honey) together in a bowl.
- Cover and place in the refrigerator.
- Include fruit before serving.
- Include milk if the mix is too thick.

Immediate Polenta With Sesame Seeds

Ingredients

- 3/4 cup instant polenta or cornmeal
- 3 cups whole milk
- 3 tablespoon. brown sugar
- 1 tsp. orange extract
- 1/2 tsp. vanilla extract
- Salt to taste
- 1 tablespoon. sesame seeds

Preparation

- Bring the milk to a boil.
- Add the polenta or cornmeal and whisk intensely to avoid lumps.
- Cook until creamy.

- Include the vanilla, salt, and sugar, and orange extract just before serving.
- Serve in a bowl and sprinkle with sesame seeds.

Calm Carrot Salad

Ingredients

- 1 pound. carrots (peeled, trimmed, and grated)
- 1/4 lb. mesclun greens
- 2 tablespoon. raisins
- 2 tablespoon. orange juice
- 1 tsp. Dr.ied oregano
- 2 tablespoon. brown sugar
- 2 tsp. olive oil
- 1/4 tsp. salt

Preparation

- In a bowl, mix the raisins, orange juice, oregano, brown sugar, olive oil, and salt. Let sit for about 5 minutes.
- Pour the Dr.essing over the carrots and mix thoroughly.
- Season with extra salt, as needed.
- Serve over mesclun leaves.

Black Bean and Cilantro Soup

Ingredients

- 8 oz. canned black beans
- 1 pint of chicken stock
- 1/2 cup fresh cilantro
- Salt to taste
- 1 tablespoon. nonfat sour cream

Preparation

- Bring the chicken stock to a boil. Include the beans, cilantro, and salt.
- Cook 30 minutes on low heat
- Blend with a hand mixer to the preferred consistency.
- Seasoning, as needed.
- Serve in a soup bowl and garnish with 1 tsp: nonfat sour cream and a sprig of cilantro.

Flavorful Cantaloupe Gazpacho

Ingredients

- 1 lb. (2 cups) cantaloupe (skin eliminated, seeded, cut into 1-inch pieces).
- 2 tablespoon.brown sugar or agave sugar.
- 2 tablespoon.port red wine.
- A dusting of fine-grated nutmeg.
- Directions.

- Mix the sugar, port, and cantaloupe. Location in the freezer for about 4 hours.
- Mix in a mixer.
- Complete with the cleaning of nutmeg.
- Serve right away in a shot glass or small cup.

Velvety Hummus

Ingredients

- 1 can (19 oz.) canned chickpeas (Dr.ained pipes and washed two times)
- 1 cup of chicken stock
- 2 tbsp. olive oil
- 1/4 tsp. sesame oil
- 1/2 tsp. salt

Preparation

- Location the chickpeas in a food mill and add the chicken stock, olive oil, sesame oil, and salt.
- Process until smooth.
- Include chicken stock as needed.
- Serve cold with toast points, oven-toasted corn chips, or small wedges of flatbread.

Watermelon and Ginger Granite

Active ingredients

- 3 cups seedless watermelon juice (combined)
- 1 cup of water
- 1/2 cup honey
- 1 entire clove
- 1 pinch ground nutmeg
- 1 tsp. fresh ginger
- 1 tsp. salt
- 1/2 tsp. lemon enthusiasm

Preparation

- Bring the water, honey, clove, nutmeg, ginger, salt, and lemon enthusiasm to a boil. Enable to cool, then strain.
- Include the syrup to the watermelon juice.
- Location the juice in a bowl that can be put in the freezer, and freeze 3 hours, Stir every 15 minutes with a sauce whisk

Quick Banana Sorbet

Ingredients

- 3 bananas, peeled
- 1 tablespoon.ginger (peeled and grated fine)
- 1/8 tsp. ground cardamom
- 2 tablespoon. honey

- 1/4 tsp. salt
- 3 cups ice

Instructions

- Location the bananas, ginger, cardamom, honey, and salt in the blender.
- 2, Blend on high until smooth.
- Include ice and mix until creamy. Include more ice as needed.
- Serve immediately or shop in the freezer.

Savoury Lentils with Texmati Brown Rice

Ingredients

- 1 lb of organic lentils (2 Â 1/2 cups), rinsed
- 8 cups water or stock
- 1 onion, chopped
- 3 cloves of garlic, sliced
- 2 carrots, sliced
- 2 stalks celery, sliced
- 1 bay leaf.
- 2 sprigs of thyme or Â 1/2 tsp Dr.ied
- Organic Texmati brown rice (follow instructions on bundle)

Direction

- Add other ingredients. Prepare up until tender (about 20 to 30 minutes), stirring sometimes and adding more liquid as needed. Season with salt and newly ground black pepper to taste.

- Frozen shrimp and veggies.

Served over millet, wild rice or quinoa

Ingredients

- 3 tbsp Canola oil
- 1lb. raw medium peeled shrimp
- 2 cups broccoli florets
- 2 cups sliced mushrooms
- 4 scallions, trimmed and chopped
- 2 tablespoon Garlic, minced
- 2 tablespoon fresh ginger, minced
- 1 cup cold veggie broth (see recipe above), combined with 2tbsps, cornstarch
- 1 plan of natural millet

Directions

- Into a hot wok or pan put oil until just cigarette smoking.
- Include veggies and stir continuously to prepare al dente.

- Add shrimp and continue to stir till simply turning pink.
- Include broth and cover for a number of minutes till shrimp is practically done.
- Uncover and add cornstarch mixture, stir until thickened and turn off the heat.
- Serve over millet cooked according to package guidelines.
- Season to taste with tamari light soy sauce

Keep in mind: This meal should be done really quickly, as you do not desire to overcook the shrimp or the vegetables. You may replace brown rice instead

LUNCH

Tuna Salad Lettuce Wraps

Components

- 1 bunch of bib lettuce
- 2 little cans (5 oz) of tuna
- 1/2 cup of mayo
- 2 sticks of celery (sliced)
- 2 Tbs. chopped sweet pickles
- pinch of salt and pepper to taste

Instructions

Wash the lettuce with cool water and let Dr.y. In a bowl, mix together the tuna, mayo, celery, pickles and salt and pepper. Lay the lettuce leaf in your hand and fill the middle with 2 Tbs.

Heartburn-Friendly Tomato Sauce-Free Lasagna

Components

- 12 ounces wide lasagna noodles
- 12 ounces very lean ground beef (ground round or ground sirloin)
- Nonstick cooking spray
- 1/2 cup low-sodium beef broth
- 1/4 cup low-fat cream cheese
- 1 1/4 cups skim milk or 1% milk, divided
- 1 tablespoon all-purpose flour
- 2 tablespoons butter or margarine
- 1/2 cup shredded good-quality Parmesan cheese
- Salt and newly ground pepper
- 1 1/2 cups grated skim mozzarella cheese

Preparation

- Heat oven to 375 F. Put a large pot of salted water on to boil and cook the lasagna noodles simply till tender. Dr.ain well.

- In a large bowl, add the browned beef and beef broth. Toss together.
- In a small blending bowl, integrate cream cheese, 1/4 cup milk, and flour. Beat till well blended. Slowly pour in staying 1 cup skim milk and beat until smooth to produce the sauce.
- Melt butter in a big, nonstick pan over medium heat. Add the milk-cream cheese mixture and continue to heat, stirring continuously, till the sauce has actually thickened about 4 minutes.
- Stir in Parmesan cheese, including salt and pepper to taste.
- Spread 1 cup of the low-fat Alfredo sauce on the bottom of a 13x9-inch baking pan. Include 3 strips of lasagna noodles and spread out half the beef mixture on top.
- Put down another 3 strips of lasagna noodles. Spread the staying beef mixture on top and set the remaining 3 strips of lasagna noodles.
- Spread out the really top with staying 1 cup low-fat Alfredo sauce. Sprinkle with mozzarella cheese and bake for 25 to 35 minutes until bubbly and golden.

Low-Fat Shrimp With Pasta

Active ingredients

- Nonstick veggie cooking spray
- 1 tablespoon olive oil
- 2 teaspoons Dr.ied basil
- 1/2 teaspoon salt
- 1 teaspoon Dr.ied oregano
- 1 pound medium shrimp, peeled and deveined (see note listed below)
- 8 ounces uncooked angel hair pasta
- 1/2 cup grated
- Parmesan cheese

Preparation

- Set a pot of water to boil for the pasta.
- Gently coat a large frying pan with nonstick veggie cooking spray. Place over medium-high heat, and add olive oil. Let heat for 1 to 2 minutes.
- Add Dr.ied basil, salt, Dr.ied oregano, and shrimp. Toss to coat shrimp with herbs and cook 6 to 8 minutes, or up until shrimp are cooked and turn pink, turning once.
- On the other hand, prepare the pasta according to package directions. Dr.ain.
- Toss shrimp mix with hot pasta.
- Sprinkle with Parmesan cheese and serve.

Heartburn-Friendly Baked Chicken Parmesan

Active ingredients

- 4 boneless, skinless chicken breasts
- 1/2 cup seasoned bread crumbs
- 3 tablespoons grated good-quality Parmesan cheese
- Dash of Italian flavouring
- Dash of salt
- 4 teaspoons olive oil

Preparation

- Heat oven to 375 F.
- Lightly coat a baking meal with veggie cooking spray.
- In a small bowl, integrate 1/2 cup skilled bread crumbs, 3 tablespoons grated good-quality Parmesan cheese (not the things in a can), a dash of Italian seasoning, and a dash of salt. Mix well.
- Lay 4 boneless, skinless chicken breasts that have been patted Dr.y on a plate and coat them with 4 teaspoons olive oil.
- Dr.edge chicken breasts on both sides in the bread-crumb mix. Transfer to the baking dish.
- Spray any staying breadcrumb mix over the chicken.
- Bake uncovered for 35 to 45 minutes, or up until done.

Salmon in Parchment with Mangoes

Active ingredients

- 1/2 cup water
- 1/4 tsp salt
- 1/2 cup brown rice
- 2sheets parchment paper (15 inches x 24 inches)
- 24-ounce salmon filets
- 1/8 tsp salt
- 1 small carrot (diced)
- 1/4 smallred bell pepper (julienned)
- 1/2 small mango (diced)
- 2/3 cup mango juice
- 2 tsp fresh marjoram (or 1 tsp. Dr.ied)
- 4 tsp unsalted butter

Direction

- In a medium saucepan, heat the water and salt. When the water boils, stir in the brown rice.
- Reduce heat to medium-low and simmer, partly covered, for about 25 - 30 minutes.
- Do not boil away all of the liquid and do not stir the rice.

- When an extremely percentage of liquid stays, remove the pan from the burner and let it stand, covered.
- Preheat the oven to 400 ° F. Fold the parchment so that it is nearly a square (15 inches x 12 inches). Starting at one end of the open edge, cut half of a heart shape in such a method that when the parchment is opened, it is in the shape of a heart.
- Wash the salmon filets in cold water and pat Dr.y. Place one salmon filet on top of each mound of rice.
- Sprinkle the 1/4 teaspoon salt evenly over the salmon filets.
- Spread the carrots, red peppers and mango over the fish uniformly.
- Sprinkle 3 tablespoons of mango juice over each the salmon. Dot the top of each fillet with 2 teaspoons of margarine.
- Close the parchment paper by rolling the edge inward starting at the point of the heart and working around to the base of the heart. The parchment pouch with the fish inside will be in the shape of a big half-circle.
- Place the pouches on a cookie sheet and after that into the oven. Minimize the heat to 375 ° F and cook for 12 minutes.
- Get rid of each pouch to a plate and let stand one minute before cutting the pouch open.

When the parchment is cut (be cautious), there will be some hot steam that escapes.

Salmon Mac and Cheese

Active ingredients

- 4 quartswater
- 8 ounces whole wheat or gluten complimentary penne pasta or shell
- 2 large eggs
- 1/2 cup2% milk
- 1/4 tsp Dried tarragon
- 4 ounces reduced-fat Monterey Jack cheese (grated)
- 8 ounces salmon (skinless; sliced into thin strips)
- 1 cup frozen pea
- 1/4 tsp salt
- fresh ground black pepper (to taste)

Direction

- Preheat the oven to 325 ° F. Place the water in a medium stock-pot over high heat and bring to a boil.

- Add the pasta and cook till the pasta is somewhat underdone. It must be not hard but slightly chewy.
- While the pasta is cooking, combine the eggs and milk in a medium blending bowl. Blend up until well mixed.
- Include the tarragon, cheese, salmon, peas, salt and pepper to the bowl and fold together.
- When the pasta is done, Dr.ain well and add it to the mixing bowl. Fold together with the cheese and salmon mixture till well combined.
- Put the mixture into a 9 inch Pyrex dish and place in the oven.
- Bake for 30 minutes.
- Let cool slightly before serving.

Salmon with Caper Mayonnaise

Active ingredients

- 1/4 cup low-fat mayonnaise
- 2 Tbsp curry parsley (minced)
- 1/2 tsp Dried tarragon
- 1 Tbsp fresh lemon juice
- 2 Tbsp capers
- 4 4 ounce salmon filets

Instructions

- Mix the mayo, parsley, tarragon, lemon juice and capers and chill.
- Preheat oven to broil. Location the salmon fillets on a non-stick cookie sheet.
- Location under broiler and cook for about 5 minutes.
- This recipe is fantastic cooked on the grill. Simply utilize a medium-hot setting on the grill and spray lightly with oil previous to cooking.
- Leading with two tablespoons of mayo and go back to broiler for another 5 minutes until the salmon is just cooked through.

Salmon with Cumin Roasted Acorn Squash

Active ingredients

- 1acorn squash (halve and seeded)
- 1/2 tsp ground cumin
- 1 tsp olive oil
- 1/4 tsp salt
- fresh ground black pepper (to taste)
- 1/4 cup Dried pumpkin seeds
- 1/16 tsp salt
- 1 tsp pure maple syrup
- spray oil
- 2 4 ounce salmon filets

Instructions

- Preheat the oven to 325 ° F. Place the squash halves in a big pan cut side down and put the pan in the preheated oven. Roast for about 40 minutes till tender. Eliminate from the oven and let cool slightly.
- Leave the oven on and place a medium frying pan inside.
- Peel the skin away from the squash. Mash the roasted squash in a bowl with the olive oil, cumin, 1/4 tsp. salt and pepper.
- While the squash is roasting, position a sheet of wax paper on the kitchen area counter.
- Place the pumpkin seeds in a non-stick frying pan over medium-high heat. Cook, stirring frequently, for about 5 minutes. See them closely and as they start to brown decrease the heat to medium.
- Add the pinch (1/16 tsp.) of salt. Prepare for about one minute more till the pumpkin seeds are browned.
- Include the maple syrup and let it bubble for about 10 seconds, shaking the pan intensely to coat the pumpkin seeds well. Eliminate the pan from the heat and stir the pumpkin seeds. Turn them out of the pan onto the wax paper to cool. Separate them from each other just after placing

on the wax paper so that they will not stick together.

- Spray the pan lightly with oil and location the salmon in the pan skin side down. Roast in the oven for about 4 minutes and turn. Roast for another 3 - 4 minutes till done.
- Serve the salmon on top of the pureed acorn squash and top with the candied pumpkin seeds.

Salmon with Parmesan Crust

Active ingredients

- 2 ounces fresh sourdough bread
- 1 ounce Parmigiano-Reggiano (grated)
- 1 clove garlic (minced)
- 1 Tbsp fresh basil (chiffonade)
- 1 tsp extra virgin olive oil
- 1/2 Tbsp balsamic vinegar
- 24-ounce salmon filets (no greater than 1/2 in. thick)
- spray olive oil

Direction

- Add the fresh sourdough bread to a food mill and process until they are fine crumbs.

- Include the parmesan, garlic, basil, olive oil and vinegar and process until the mixture is well combined. This will make a damp breadcrumb mixture.
- Put a non-stick skillet in the oven on the most affordable possible rack. Leave the pan in the oven for at least 10 minutes.
- Put the salmon fillets on a cutting board skin side down and pat the breadcrumb mixture onto the top of each fillet.
- Get rid of the skillet from the oven and gently spray with oil. Transfer the salmon filets (skin side down) to the pan and return to the oven. Cook for 6 minutes for rare.
- Turn on the broiler and broil up until the crust is golden brown (about 3 - 5 more minutes).

Seared Halibut with Basil Oil

Active ingredients

- 1/4 cup extra virgin olive oil
- 1/2 cup fresh basil leaves
- 2 4 ounce filets halibut
- 1/4 tsp salt
- fresh ground black pepper (to taste).
- spray olive oil

Direction

- Place the olive oil and basil in a blender or mini chopper and procedure until smooth.
- Preheat the oven to 425 ° F. Place a medium-sized frying pan in the oven.
- While the oven is heating up rinse the halibut filets with cold water and pat Dr.y. Place them on a cutting board skin side up. Cut shallow slits in the skin about 1/4 inch apart. Spray the skin side of the fish with the salt and pepper.
- When the oven is hot spray the pan gently with oil. Place the fish in the pan skin side down. Return the pan to the oven and cook for about 10 - 12 minutes.
- Serve the fish skin side up and top with 1 1/2 teaspoons of basil oil.

Seared Halibut with Basil Pea Puree

Active ingredients

- 1/210 ounce plan frozen peas
- 1 1/2 Tbsp fresh basil
- 1/8 tsp salt
- fresh ground black pepper
- 24-ounce fresh halibut filet
- 1/2 tsp extra virgin olive oil

Instructions

- Thaw the frozen peas and rinse under cool water. Add and Dr.ain to a mixer with the fresh basil, salt and pepper.
- Purée in a blender until smooth.
- Place in a saucepan and heat over medium heat. Heat the sauce, stirring regularly. When hot, reduce the heat to low to keep warm.
- Preheat oven to 400 ° F.
- Turn the halibut filets skin side up on a cutting board and gently cut stripes in the skin about 1 inch apart. Do not cut entirely through the skin to the flesh (this is to keep the filet from curling as the fish cooks).
- In a big non-stick frying pan, heat the olive oil over high heat. The oil should be really hot - almost cigarette smoking.
- Place the halibut fillets in the hot pan skin side up. Cook for about 2 minutes up until the flesh is light brown and has a slight crust to it.
- Allow and turn to prepare for about a minute on the skin side and after that location in the hot oven. Roast for about 8 more minutes.
- As the fish nears being done, divide the sauce in between 4 plates making a big swimming pool in the bottom of each plate. Top the sauce with the roasted fish and garnish with fresh basil sprigs.

Entire Wheat Linguine with Shrimp and Leeks

Active ingredients

- 2 quartswater
- 4 ounces whole wheat or gluten-free linguine
- 2 tsp extra virgin olive oil
- 2 large leeks (cleaned well and sliced into rounds)
- 2 Tbsp white wine vinegar
- 2 Tbsp white, red wine
- 1/2 cup low salt chicken or veggie broth
- 1 Tbsp capers
- 3/4 ounce goat cheese
- fresh ground black pepper (to taste)
- 8 ounces large shrimp (peeled and deveined)
- 2 TbspDr.ied pumpkin seeds
- 2 Tbsp fresh basil
- 2 Tbsp red bell pepper (diced)

Instructions

- Place the water in a big stockpot over high heat.
- While the water is concerning a boil location the olive oil in a big frying pan over medium-high heat. Add the leeks and cook, stirring regularly. Don't let the leeks brown too much (a little golden at the most).

- When the leeks are soft, include the linguine to the boiling water. Stir often.
- Include the vinegar, wine, chicken stock, capers, goat shrimp, pepper and cheese to the frying pan with the leeks. Increase the heat to medium-high. Cook, stirring regularly, After the sauce is simmering and the shrimp begin to turn pink decrease the heat to medium and include the pumpkin seeds.
- When the linguine is done, move it from the pasta water to the frying pan with the leeks using tongs. Let most of the linguine Dr.ain (it is OKAY to have some of the pasta water in your sauce).
- Add the basil and cook for another minute tossing to mix the pasta with the leeks and sauce.
- Serve with bell pepper on top of diced red.

Sesame Seared Whitefish with Cilantro Oil

Active ingredients

- 1 Tbsp roasted sesame oil
- 2 Tbsp low salt soy or gluten-free tamari sauce
- 1 Tbsp fresh ginger (minced)
- 1/2 tsp sugar
- 2 Tbspbeer
- fresh ground black pepper (to taste)

- 4 4 ounce halibut or other white fish fillets
- 6 tsp cilantro Oil

Direction

- Position the sesame oil, soy sauce, ginger, sugar, beer and pepper in a Pyrex dish or a Ziplock bag.
- Location the fish in the marinade and place it in the fridge. Turn the fish about every 30 minutes and marinate for at least two hours.
- Place a medium frying pan over medium-high heat. When hot, include the fish.
- Cook on the very first side for about 10 minutes and turn. Add the marinade and cook for another 7 to 10 minutes.
- Serve each filet topped with 1 1/2 teaspoons Cilantro Oil.

Basic Pan-Fried Fish

Active ingredients

- 2 large egg whites
- 4 Tbsp coarse ground cornmeal
- 1/4 tsp salt
- fresh ground black pepper (to taste)

- 4 4 ounce filets whitefish (cod, halibut, grouper, Dr.um, or catfish)
- 4 Tbsp fresh dill
- 2 tsp canola oil

Direction

- Blend egg whites up until frothy.
- Mix the cornmeal together with the salt and pepper.
- Dig up the fish in the egg white and after that spray each side with dill. Dr.edge in the cornmeal until well coated.
- When all 4 filets are covered, position a big frying pan over medium-high heat and include the oil. When the oil is hot, include the covered fish. Cook for about 6-7 minutes on each side.
- Serve topped with the Tartar Sauce of your choice.

Tuna Noodle Casserole

Active ingredients

- 3 quartswater
- 16 ounces whole wheat or gluten-free rotini pasta

- 2cans Campbell's Healthy Request Cream of Mushroom Soup
- 1/4 cup2% milk
- 26-ounce cans light tuna crammed in water (no salt added)
- 116-ounce bag of frozen peas
- fresh ground black pepper (to taste)
- 1/8 tsp ground nutmeg
- 2 ounces Parmigiano-Reggiano (grated)
- spray cooking oil

Instructions

- Preheat the oven to 375 ° F. Place the water in a medium stockpot over high heat.
- When the water boils, add the pasta and cook for ten minutes. Dr.ain pipes and reserve.
- While the pasta is cooking, place the mushroom soup, milk, tuna (Dr.ained pipes), peas, pepper and nutmeg in a large bowl. Fold together gently.
- Include the cooked pasta to the mushroom mix and fold together carefully.
- Spray a 12-inch oblong pan gently with oil. Sprinkle the cheese over the leading and put the casserole in the oven.

Whitefish in Foil with Mustard Sauce

Active ingredients

- 8 ounces red potatoes (cut into 1/4 inch dice)
- 2 tsp extra virgin olive oil
- 4 Tbsp white wine
- 2 tsp coarse ground mustard
- 1/8 tsp Dried tarragon
- 1/4 tsp salt
- 2 4 ounce cod fillets (or halibut, or grouper)
- 1 medium carrot (cut into 1/4 inch dice)
- 4 ounces snap peas
- 1/4 medium yellow bell pepper (cut into thin julienne strips)
- fresh ground black pepper (to taste)
- 2 tsp unsalted butter

Direction

- Preheat, the oven to 325 ° F., Combine the diced potatoes with the olive oil, white wine, mustard, tarragon and salt in a glass bowl. Fold together until well blended.
- Place the bowl in a microwave for 1 minute on high. Stir and remove the bowl. Repeat for another minute. Remove the bowl and stir.
- Fold 2 pieces of aluminium foil so that they are almost a square (15 inches x 12 inches). Beginning at one end of the folded edge, cut

half of a heart shape in such a method that when the foil is unfolded, it is in the shape of a heart.

- Place the potato mixture on top of one side of the heart shape for each of the pieces of foil. Leading each with the cod filets.
- Include half of the carrots, snap peas and yellow pepper strips. Leading with fresh ground black pepper and one teaspoon of butter for each fish.
- Close the foil by rolling the edge inward, beginning at the point of the heart and working around to the base of the heart. The foil pouch with the fish within will be in the shape of a large half-circle.
- Place the pouches on a cookie sheet and after that into the oven and cook for 18 minutes.
- Get rid of each pouch to a plate and let stand 30 seconds prior to cutting the pouch open. There will be some hot steam that gets away when the parchment is cut (beware!).

Whitefish with Root Vegetables in Warm Vinaigrette

Active ingredients

- 4 cups of water
- 4 ounces parsnips (peeled and cut into 1/4 inch dice)

* 2 ounces carrots (peeled and cut into 1/4 inch dice)
* 2 ounces turnip (peeled and cut into 1/4 inch dice)
* 4 tsp.extra virgin olive oil (divided)
* 2 large shallots (finely diced)
* 1 tsp, fresh thyme leaves
* 1/4lemon (juiced)
* 1/16 tsp salt (divided)
* 1 tsp coarse ground mustard
* fresh ground black pepper (to taste)
* 1 medium green onion
* 2 tsp.unsalted butter.
* 2 4 ounces filets white fish (e.g., cod, halibut)

Instructions

* Place the water in a saucepan over high heat and bring to a boil.
* Decrease the heat to simmer and add the parsnips, carrots and turnip. Simmer for 5 minutes, then get rid of to a bowl full of ice water.
* Shut off the heat however leave the pan with the water on the stove.
* Place a little skillet over medium-high heat.
* Add 1 teaspoon of the olive oil to the pan, swirl, and after that add the shallot and thyme.

- Cook for about 10 minutes, stirring periodically, till the shallot is clear.
- While the shallots are cooking, place 2 teaspoons olive oil with the lemon juice, 1/8 teaspoon salt, mustard, and pepper and whisk together.
- Cut the green complement of the green onion and thinly slice crosswise.
- Cut the white part of the green onion lengthwise in half and then slice lengthwise in half once again. Thinly slice the white part crosswise.
- Add the white and green part of the green onion to the meal with the vinaigrette.
- When the shallots are done, add them to the dish with the vinaigrette and toss carefully till blended.
- Turn the heat back on high for the water in the saucepan.
- Place a medium frying pan over high heat with 1 teaspoon olive oil and 2 teaspoons butter.
- When the butter is hot, add the fish and sauté for about 5 to 6 minutes.
- Turn and prepare for another 4 to 5 minutes.
- While the fish is cooking, add the cooled veggies to warm water and reheat for about 3 minutes.
- Dr.ain and add the veggies to the vinaigrette and toss till well blended.

- Divide the veggies in between 2 plates and leading with the prepared fish. Leading with 2 tablespoons of the Onion Confit and serve.

Blue Cheese Crab and Fusilli Pasta

Active ingredients

- 1 Tbsp olive oil
- 1 large white onion
- 1/4 cup white wine
- 1/2 cup water
- 1/2 cup low sodium chicken or veggie broth
- 1/2 tsp lemon enthusiasm
- 1-ounce blue cheese
- 4 quartswater
- 8 ounces carrots
- 4 ounces whole-wheat fusilli pasta
- 8 ounces lump crabmeat
- 1 Tbsp flat-leaf parsley

Active ingredients for Fusilli Pasta

- 1 Tbsp olive oil
- 1 large white onion
- 1/4 cup white red wine
- 1/2 cup water
- 1/2 cup low sodium chicken or veggie broth
- 1/2 tsp lemon zest
- 1-ounce blue cheese

- 4 quartswater
- 8 ounces carrots
- 4 ounces whole-wheat fusilli pasta
- 8 ounces lump crabmeat
- 1 Tbsp flat-leaf parsley

Instructions

- Place the olive oil in a medium-sized stainless steel saucepan over medium heat. Include the onion. Cook, stirring frequently, for about 10 minutes. Do not let the onions brown.
- As the onions start to turn a shiny milky white colour, include the Gewurztraminer, water, chicken stock, salt and lemon passion.
- Cook for about 15 minutes, up until the onions are softened. Use a mixer or stick blender and puree till smooth. Return the sauce to the pan and add the blue cheese. Reduce the heat to very low and stir until the cheese melts and the sauce is smooth.
- Place the water in a big saucepan over high heat and bring to a boil. Add the matchstick carrots and cook for about 3 minutes up until a little tender. Eliminate with a slotted spoon to a paper towel.

- While the water is still boiling, add the pasta. Cook, stirring periodically, for about 10 - 12 minutes up until the pasta is tender.
- While the pasta is cooking include the crabmeat to the sauce and reheat carefully.
- When the pasta is done, Dr.ain thoroughly and contribute to the sauce. Toss together with the carrots and parsley and serve.

Crab Cakes

Ingredients

- 1 lb lump crabmeat
- 1/3 cup low-sodium saltine crackers
- 1/2 tsp tabasco sauce
- 2 tsp Worcestershire sauce
- 1 Tbsp shallot (minced)
- 2 tsp dijon mustard
- 1 large egg white
- 1rib celery (diced)
- 1 Tbsp fresh lemon juice
- 2 Tbsp reduced-fat mayonnaise
- 1/8 tsp salt
- pepper
- 2 tsp extra virgin olive oil

Instructions

- Choose over crabmeat getting rid of any shell.
- Break the crackers into about 1/4 inch pieces.
- Fold the crabmeat together with the crumbled saltines. Add Tabasco sauce, Worcestershire sauce, shallot, mustard, egg white, celery, lemon juice, pepper, salt and mayo.
- Fold together gently until well combined. Be careful to not separate the crabmeat excessive.
- Kind into 8 cakes and chill. This can be made up to 12 hours in advance.
- Preheat the oven to 400 ° F.
- Place the oil in a big non-stick skillet over high heat until the oil is practically smoking.
- Place cakes in the hot oil and cook over medium-high heat for about 3 minutes up until brown. Cook and turn for about 2 minutes. Place in the hot oven. Prepare for another 9-- 10 minutes.

Pecan Shrimp Linguine

Ingredients

- 8 ounces crimini mushrooms (sliced)
- 3 quartswater
- 4 ounces spinach linguine
- 2 tsp olive oil
- 1/4 cup raw pecans (sliced coarsely)
- 1 tsp Dried rosemary

- 8 ounces shrimp (peeled and deveined)
- 2 Tbsp all-purpose flour
- 1/2 cup2% milk
- 1/4 tsp salt
- fresh ground black pepper (to taste)

Direction

- Place a large non-stick skillet over medium-high heat. Add the mushrooms and cook, tossing frequently, for about 15 minutes. Let the mushrooms brown entirely and then remove to a plate.
- While the mushrooms are cooking location the water in a large saucepan over high heat. When it is boiling, include the linguine. Stir often.
- While the pasta is cooking location a large non-stick skillet over medium-high heat. Add the olive oil and pecans and cook, stirring frequently. Let the pecans brown but if they are cooking too quickly, turn the heat to medium.
- When the pecans are brown, add the rosemary and shrimp. Cook, tossing regularly, for about 5 minutes. Spray the flour over the shrimp and toss until it is well integrated. Prepare for another 2 minutes.

- Include the milk and salt. Prepare till the sauce begins to thicken. Dr.ain pipes the pasta scheduling about a half cup of the pasta water.
- Include the linguine to the shrimp and sauce and toss. If the sauce is too thick, add some of the pasta water 2 tablespoons at a time. Serve.

Saffron Scallops Carbonara

Ingredients

- 1/8 tsp saffron threads
- 3 quartswater
- 4 ounces whole wheat or gluten-free linguine
- 2 tsp olive oil
- 2 cloves garlic (gently crushed)
- 1-ounce prosciutto (diced)
- 1 cup frozen pea (thawed)
- 6 ounces scallops (cut into quarters)
- 2 large eggs
- 1 ounce Parmigiano-Reggiano (grated)
- fresh ground black pepper (to taste)

Direction

- Place the saffron in a little bowl or teacup.
- Pour the water in a big saucepan over high heat.
- When the water boils, remove 1/4 cup and put over the saffron.

- Add the pasta to the pot with the boiling water. Let cook for about 12 minutes till almost done.
- When the pasta is practically done, place the olive oil in a medium frying pan over medium heat. Add the garlic and prosciutto.
- Cook, stirring regularly, till the ham begins to turn crisp. Change the heat so that the garlic does not turn dark brown but light golden.
- Add the scallops and peas and reduce the heat to low.
- When the pasta is prepared, add the saffron/water mixture to the frying pan and then the pasta. Increase the heat to medium-high.
- Blend the eggs together with the grated parmesan. Season with pepper.
- After the pasta is hot (about 2 minutes), dispose of the garlic and add the egg and cheese mixture to the skillet.
- Fold together well with a rubber spatula to cook the eggs. Serve right away.

Scallops Gratin

Ingredients

- 1slice entire wheat or gluten-free bread
- 1/2 tsp Dried basil

- 1/4 tsp Dried marjoram
- 1/8 tsp Dried tarragon
- 1 tsp olive oil
- spray olive oil
- 12 ounces crimini or button mushrooms (quartered)
- 1 tsp function flour
- 1/4 cup low sodium chicken or vegetable broth
- 1/4 tsp salt
- fresh ground black pepper (to taste)
- 1 tsp unsalted butter
- 12 ounces sea scallops
- 2 ounces fontina cheese (shredded)

Instructions

- Toast the slice of whole wheat bread until golden brown.
- Place the bread in a mixer or small chopper and add the basil, marjoram, tarragon and olive oil. Process until great bread crumbs.
- Preheat the oven to 325 ° F. Spray a big non-stick pan with olive oil. Place the pan over medium-high heat and include the mushrooms. Cook, tossing often, for about 10 - 15 minutes till the mushrooms are well caramelized.
- Include the chicken stock and the salt. Cook up until the sauce begins to thicken and add the butter.

- Dr.y and clean the pan and location over medium-high heat. Spray with olive oil and after the pan is hot add the sea scallops. Cook for about 2 minutes on each side until seared light brown.
- Put the seared scallops into 2 au gratin or other shallow ovenproof dishes. Top each meal with half of the mushroom mix and after that half of the bread crumbs.
- Place in the preheated oven and cook for about 12 minutes (depending on the size of the private scallops). Leading with the cheese and cook for another 2 minutes till the cheese is melted. Serve.

Lentil and Chickpea Soup

Ingredients

- 2 quartswater
- 4 ouncesDr.ied lentils
- 4 ouncesDr.ied chickpeas
- 2 tsp.olive oil
- 4 ounces celery (diced) (about 3 stalks)
- 4 ounces carrots (peeled and diced) (about 2 medium carrots)
- 3 cups no salt included veggie stock
- 1 cup of water
- 1/4 tsp salt

- 3bay leaves
- to taste fresh ground black pepper

Direction

- Place the water, lentils, and chickpeas in a big bowl and let mean a minimum of 10 hours.
- Dr.ain and wash. Reserve.
- Pour the olive oil in a large saucepan over medium-high heat.
- Include the celery and cook for about 4 minutes up until slightly translucent. Stir often.
- Include the carrots and cook for about 3 minutes. Stir frequently.
- Include the veggie stock, water, bay leaves, and the lentils and chickpeas.
- Minimize the heat to medium-low and simmer for 45 minutes.
- Include the salt and pepper and simmer for another 15 minutes.
- Serve.

Potage a la Florentine

Ingredients

- 1-ounce unsalted butter
- 1/2 cup onions (minced)

- 1 lb frozen spinach
- 4 Tbsp all-purpose flour
- 4 cups low sodium chicken or veggie broth
- 2 cups of water
- 1/2 cup brown rice (uncooked)
- 1 tsp ground nutmeg
- 1/2 tsp salt
- 1/4 cup sherry
- 2 cups2% milk

Instructions

- Melt the butter in a medium stockpot over medium heat. Cook the onions in butter till soft then include spinach and cook till hot.
- Add flour gradually so as not to clump and cook for two minutes over low heat.
- Include the chicken stock and heat slowly. The soup will thicken.
- Add rice and cook up until tender.
- If the soup is too thick), include sherry, nutmeg and salt and cook for 3 minutes (include water.
- Puree with a stick mixer (or in multiple batches in a mixer). Transfer back to the pot. Reheat carefully while including the milk.

Turkey White Bean Soup

Ingredients

- 2 quartswater
- leftover turkey bones
- 2 lbs of leftover turkey meat
- 3 15 ounces can no salt added white beans (Dr.ained pipes and rinsed)
- 3 large ribs celery (thickly sliced)
- 3 large carrots (peeled and cut into large chunks)
- 3/4 tsp salt
- fresh ground black pepper (to taste)
- 1 TbspDr.ied sage

Instructions

- Place the water in a big stockpot over high heat. Add the turkey bones, and when the water simply begins to boil decrease the heat to simmer. Simmer for 30 minutes.
- Pressure and discard the bones. Include the broth to the pot with the turkey meat, white beans, celery, carrots, pepper, sage and salt.
- Simmer over medium heat for about 90 minutes. Serve.

Roasted Eggplant Soup

Active ingredients

- 1/2 lb plum tomatoes (cut in half)
- 1 1/2 lbs eggplant (quartered lengthwise)
- 1/2 lb shallots (peeled and halved)
- 6 cloves garlic (peeled)
- spray olive oil
- 1 tsp dried thyme
- 3 1/2 cups low salt chicken or vegetable broth
- 1/2 cup white wine
- 2 cups of water
- 1/4 tsp salt
- 1 cup2% of milk

Instructions

- Preheat oven to 400 ° F.
- Place vegetables in a big roasting pan. Spray lightly with olive oil. Roast up until tender and brown in spots (about 45 minutes).
- Include the roasted veggies, thyme, chicken stock, white, red wine and water to the pot and place over medium-high heat. Add 4 cups chicken stock and bring to boil.

- Reduce heat to medium-low and simmer till vegetables hurt (about 45 minutes). Cool slightly.
- Puree with a stick blender the veggies and salt until smooth (or in multiple batches in a blender). Return soup to saucepan.

Iced Cucumber Soup

Ingredients

- 1 tsp unsalted butter
- 3 large cucumbers (peeled, seeded and sliced)
- 2 cups low sodium chicken or vegetable broth
- 1/2 cup white wine
- 1 Tbsp fresh dill
- 1/2 tsp salt
- 1/8 tsp coarsely ground pepper
- dash ground nutmeg
- 3/4 cup-fat sour cream
- 1/2 cup-fat yoghurt
- very finely sliced cucumber
- fresh dill

Instructions

- Melt the butter in a big non-stick skillet over medium heat. Include the cucumber and sauté for about 10 minutes. The cucumber must be gently browned.

- Add the chicken broth and increase heat to medium-high. Bring the soup to a boil, stirring occasionally, and add the white wine.
- Lower the heat to medium and simmer for about ten minutes stirring often. Add pepper, dill and salt.
- Decrease the heat to medium-low and simmer two minutes.
- (Or pour 1/2 of the soup in a mixer jar and blend on melt until smooth. Repeat with the other half of the soup and enable it to cool.).
- After the soup is cooled add 1/2 cup of the sour cream and the yoghurt to the soup. Whisk till smooth and after that cover and chill till really cold.
- To serve, ladle into private bowls, leading each with a dollop of the staying sour cream. Garnish with cucumber pieces and fresh dill.

Beef Tips in Brown Gravy - GERD Friendly Version

Active ingredients

- 2 quarts ice water
- 2 lbs onions (sliced)
- 3 tsp olive oil

- 1 lb button mushroom (sliced)
- 1 lb top round or other lean beef (cut into 1/2 inch strips)
- 1 1/4 cup water (divided)
- 1/2 tsp salt
- fresh ground black pepper (to taste)
- 1 TbspWorcestershire sauce
- 3 quartswater
- 8 ounces whole wheat or gluten-free spaghetti
- 1 Tbsp cornstarch

Instructions

- Soak the chopped onions in 2 quarts ice water for 45 minutes and after that Dr.ain.
- Pour 2 teaspoons of olive oil in a big skillet over high heat. Add the mushrooms and cook for about 10 minutes, tossing regularly.
- When the mushrooms are browned and well caramelized, eliminate them to a plate. Include 1 teaspoon olive oil to the pan and then the chopped onions. Cook, stirring often, up until well browned.
- Include the beef and cook until browned.
- Include the prepared mushrooms, 1 cup water, salt, pepper and Worcestershire sauce. Stir and cover. Reduce the heat to medium-low and simmer for about 30 minutes. Stir periodically.

- After about 20 minutes of cooking location, the water in a medium stockpot over high heat. When the water is boiling, add the pasta. Cook for about 12 minutes till done.
- When the pasta is ready to serve, location 1/4 cup cold water in a small meal with the cornstarch. Include the mix to the pan with the beef.
- Dr.ain the pasta and serve topped with the beef tips and gravy.

Chicken Fried Steak

Ingredients

- 1 cup salt included chicken stock
- 1 tsp Dried rosemary
- 4 4 ounce top sirloin or bottom round filets
- 1 large egg
- 1 cup bread crumbs, panko crumbs, or gluten-free panko crumbs
- 2 Tbsp-fat buttermilk
- 1/4 tsp salt
- fresh ground black pepper (to taste)
- 2 Tbsp canola oil
- 1/2 cup2% milk
- 4 tsp cornstarch

Direction

- Place the chicken stock in a small saucepan with the rosemary. Place over high heat, give a boil and reduce the heat to a simmer. Reduce the chicken stock by about half. Get rid of from the heat and let cool.
- Utilizing a fulfil tenderizer or mallet, pound the filets lightly until they are a little flattened.
- Whisk together the egg and buttermilk.
- Place the breadcrumbs on a plate.
- Dig up the beef filets in the egg mix. Cover well.
- Place the filets on the plate with the breadcrumbs.
- Sprinkle with 1/4 teaspoon of the pepper and the salt.
- Turn the filets over to coat the other side of the filets. Pat to coat the filets well with the breadcrumbs.
- Place the oil in a large skillet over medium-high heat.
- When the pan is hot, include the breaded filets. Prepare on the very first side for about 8 minutes.
- While the steaks are cooking, include the cornstarch to the cold milk and stir well with a fork up until mixed.
- Turn the steaks and cook for another 8 minutes or until the breadcrumbs are well browned.

- Eliminate the steaks to a warm plate.
- Put the chicken stock through a strainer (to eliminate the Dr.ied rosemary) into the hot frying pan. Whisk well.
- Let the stock reduce by about 1/3. Include the milk and cornstarch and blend continually over medium heat up until the sauce is thickened.
- Serve the steak topped with the sauce.

Cookout Burgers

Ingredients

- 1 lb95% lean ground beef
- 1/4 tsp salt
- 2 tsp dijon mustard
- 2 tsp Worcestershire sauce
- 1/2 tsp garlic powder
- fresh ground black pepper (to taste)

Instructions

- In a non-reactive bowl, blend together the salt, mustard, Worcestershire, garlic powder, and pepper.
- Include the ground beef and mix completely.
- Pat the hamburger into 4 4-ounce patties.

- Place a non-stick pan over medium-high heat. When the pan is heated, put the burgers in the pan.
- For medium-rare burgers, cook 4-5 minutes, then turn over and prepare for another 4-5 minutes. (Adjust time as required for the desired doneness.).
- Serve on hamburger buns with accompaniments of your choice.

Flank Steak with Blackberry Glaze

Ingredients

- 2 Tbspblackberry preserves.
- 1 Tbsp light brown sugar
- 4 Tbsp white wine
- 1/2 tsp lemon enthusiasm
- 1/4 tsp salt
- fresh ground black pepper (to taste)
- 1/8 tsp Dried marjoram leaves
- spray olive oil
- 1 lb crimini (or other wild) mushrooms (quartered)
- 1 tsp olive oil
- 8 ounces flank steak
- 2 tsp unsalted butter

Instructions

- Preheat the oven to 375 ° F. Place a big skillet in the oven.
- Integrate the blackberry preserves with the brown sugar, 2 tablespoons of the wine, lemon enthusiasm, marjoram, pepper and salt. Stir well till blended.
- Spray the pan in the oven lightly with olive oil. Add the quartered mushrooms. Roast the mushrooms for about 20 minutes. Shake the pan occasionally. Cook till the mushrooms are well caramelized.
- Eliminate the mushrooms from the pan and reserve. Add the olive oil to the pan. Return the skillet to the oven and increase the temperature to 425 ° F
- . When the oven is hot, include the flank steak to the pan. Spoon about 1/3 of the blackberry sauce over the top of the steak. Cook for about 6 minutes and turn. Top the steak with the rest of the sauce. Cook for another 5 - 7 minutes and eliminate the pan from the oven. Set the steak on a cutting board to rest.
- Place the pan on the stove over medium heat. Include the mushrooms to the pan with the butter and the remaining 2 tablespoons of the

red wine. Stir well as the butter melts and reduce the heat to low.

- Slice the steak and location the slices on plates. Leading with the mushrooms and sauce. Serve.

Kung Pao Beef - GERD/ Acid Reflux Friendly Version

Active ingredients

- 16 ounces flank steak (cut into 1-inch cubes)
- 2 tsp low-sodium soy sauce or gluten-free tamari sauce
- 2 tsp sake or sweet Gewurztraminer
- 1 tsp sesame oil
- 2 tsp rice vinegar
- 2 tsp honey
- 1 tsp cornstarch
- 2 cups of water
- 1 cup jasmine rice
- 1 Tbsp sesame oil
- 1inch ginger root (peeled and minced)
- 2 Tbsp rice vinegar
- 2 Tbsp low-sodium soy sauce or gluten-free tamari sauce
- 3/4 cup water
- 1/4 cup Dried roasted peanuts (sliced coarsely)

Direction

- Place the 2 teaspoons low-sodium soy sauce, sake, 1 teaspoon sesame oil, rice vinegar, honey and cornstarch in a bowl and stir until well mixed. Add the flank steak cubes and toss-up until layered. Place the bowl in the refrigerator.
- While the beef is marinating place the water in a medium saucepan over high heat. When the water boils, stir in the jasmine rice.
- Minimize heat to medium-low and simmer, partly covered, for about 25 - 30 minutes.
- Do not boil away all of the liquid and do not stir the rice.
- When a real percentage of liquid remains, get rid of the pan from the burner and let it stand, covered, for 5 minutes prior to serving.
- Include the sesame oil and heat for a few moments. Minimize the heat to medium and add the ginger. Prepare for about one minute.
- Add the beef and cook for about one minute till browned on the outside.
- Add the rice vinegar and soy sauce. Cook the beef, tossing frequently. When the beef is almost done, include the water and stir till well mixed. When the beef is prepared through serve over the rice and top with the peanuts.

Meatballs

Ingredients

- 1 lb extra lean beef (7% fat)
- 2 ounces fresh bread crumbs
- 1 tsp dried oregano
- 1 tsp Dried basil
- 1 tsp Dried rosemary
- 1 tsp dried thyme
- 1/2 tsp salt
- 1/8 tsp fresh ground black pepper
- spray olive oil

Instructions

- Preheat oven to 400 ° F. Place a large non-stick frying pan in the oven.
- Mix the hamburger together with the bread crumbs, oregano, basil, rosemary, thyme, salt and pepper until well mixed.
- Roll the mixture into a large ball and cut in half. Roll each into two balls and cut each of those in half.
- Spray the hot frying pan lightly with olive oil. Place the meatballs in the frying pan and go back to the oven. Prepare for about 12-- 15 minutes till they are firm to touch.

Healthy Meatloaf

Active ingredients

- 1 lb extra lean hamburger
- 4 ounces fresh bread crumbs
- 1 tsp dried oregano
- 1 tsp Dried basil
- 1 tsp Dried rosemary
- 1 tsp dried thyme
- 1/2 tsp salt
- 1/8 tsp fresh ground black pepper
- 3/4 cup tomato sauce

Instructions

- Preheat oven to 325 ° F. Line an elongate Pyrex dish or large frying pan with aluminium foil.
- Mix the ground beef together with the bread crumbs, oregano, basil, rosemary, thyme, salt and pepper up until well mixed.
- Roll the mixture into a big ball and after that shape into a loaf. Location, the loaf in the aluminium foil, lined pan. Continue to shape up until the loaf is firm by pushing it together.
- Place the pan in the oven. Cook for about 30 minutes and leading with the marinara sauce. Go back to the oven and cook for about 20 minutes up until the internal temperature is 150 ° F. Remove from the oven and let rest for about 5-- 10 minutes before slicing.

Roast Leg of Lamb

Ingredients

- 2 lb boneless leg of lamb
- 3 Tbsp fresh oregano
- 1/2 tsp salt
- fresh ground black pepper (to taste)
- 1 tsp olive oil
- 1/2 cup low sodium chicken broth
- 1 Tbsp unsalted butter

Direction

- Preheat the oven to 325 ° F. Carefully cut the excess fat and silverskin from the outside of the leg of lamb.
- Sprinkle the within the leg with the oregano leaves, 1/4 teaspoon of the salt and pepper. Roll the leg up and truss using kitchen twine.
- Pour the olive oil in a large frying pan over medium-high heat. When the oil is hot, include the lamb.
- Roast the lamb for about 45 minutes. Turn every 15 minutes to brown each side of the lamb.
- The very best way to look for the lamb being done is utilizing a meat thermometer. When it

checks out 145 ° F, remove from the oven and set the roast on a plate to rest. (Alternatively, the roast will take about 75 minutes to prepare.).

- Place the frying pan over medium-high heat and include the chicken broth. Include the remaining 1/4 teaspoon salt and whisk as the sauce reduces by about half. Add the butter and blend till melted.
- Serve the lamb sliced with the sauce.

Pork Chops with Savory Apple Compote

Active ingredients

- 2 tsp olive oil (divided)
- 1 small shallot (minced)
- 1 medium rib celery (small dice)
- 1apple (peeled and cut into medium dice)
- 1/4 cup white red wine
- 1/2 cup water
- 3/4 tsp salt (divided)
- fresh ground black pepper (to taste)
- 1 tsp paprika
- 1/4 tsp ground cumin
- 1/8 tsp ground cinnamon
- 1 tsp maple syrup
- 4 4 ounce boneless centre-cut pork chops

Direction

- Place a large pan in the oven and heat the oven to 375F.
- Pour1 teaspoon olive oil in a medium saucepan over medium heat. Add the shallot and sauté for about 2 minutes.
- Add the celery and continue sautéing for another two minutes, then include the apple and continue sautéing for another two minutes.
- Add the water, white wine, salt, pepper, paprika, cumin, cinnamon and maple syrup and stir.
- Simmer 20 minutes.
- While simmering, place 1 teaspoon of olive oil in the pan in the oven. Add the pork chops, sprinkle 1/8 teaspoon salt over the pork chops, and return the pan to the oven.
- Prepare for 8 minutes, then turn the chops over and cook for another 7 minutes or till the centre reaches 140 degrees. Serve topped with the compote.

Pork Chops with Bourbon Pecan Sauce

Active ingredients

- 1 tsp olive oil
- 1/2 cup chopped pecans
- 3/4 cup low sodium chicken or veggie broth
- 1/4 cup bourbon

* 1 tsp rubbed sage (or 1 Tbsp. fresh sage, chopped)
* 1/2 tsp salt
* 4 tsp light brown sugar
* spray oil
* 44-ounce centre cut pork chops (boneless)

Instructions

* Pour the olive oil in a small saucepan over medium heat. Add the pecans and cook slowly, stirring often. Do not allow the pecans to burn.
* After the pecans have browned somewhat, add the chicken stock, bourbon, sage, salt and brown sugar. Decrease the heat to medium-low and simmer the sauce, swirling frequently. Minimize by about 1/3.
* While the sauce is decreasing, pre-heat the oven to 375 ° F. Place a large frying pan in the oven.
* When the sauce is minimized, turn the heat to low.
* Spray the preheated skillet gently with oil and include the pork chops in the pan. Return the pan to the oven and cook for about 7 -8 minutes on the first side. Turn and cook for another 7 - 10 minutes up until done.
* Serve topped with about 3 tablespoons of sauce.

Pork Chops with Herbed Butter - Coumadin Safe Version

Active ingredients

- 3 Tbsp fresh herbs, such as basil, rosemary, tarragon, sage, thyme - NOT parsley (minced)
- 3 Tbsp unsalted butter
- 1/4 tsp salt
- 1/2 tsp honey
- spray olive oil
- fresh ground black pepper
- 24-ounce centre cut pork chops

Instructions

- Mince the herbs and blend them together with the spread, salt and honey. This can be done up to 24 hours beforehand and kept in the refrigerator.
- Preheat oven to 425 ° F. Place a large skillet in the oven.
- Return the pan to the oven and cook for about 7 minutes and then turn. Cook for another 7 to 10 minutes and serve topped with 1/2 of the herbed butter for each pork slice.

DINNER

Heartburn-Friendly Chicken Pot Pie

Active ingredients

- 1 pound boneless, skinless chicken breasts
- 1/2 teaspoon salt
- 1 tablespoon olive oil
- 1 cup frozen carrots, defrosted and Dr.ained
- 1 cup frozen peas, thawed and Dr.ained pipes
- 1 (14.75-ounce) can cream-style corn
- 3/4 cup skim milk, divided into 1/4 cup and 1/2 cup portions
- 1 cup biscuit mix

Preparation

- Heat oven to 400 degrees F.
- Cut chicken breasts into 1-inch cubes and season with 1/2 teaspoon salt.
- Heat 1 tablespoon olive oil or grease in a frying pan over medium-high heat.
- Add the 1 pound of salted chicken breast cubes and cook for 8 minutes, stirring occasionally, or until browned.
- Place chicken into a 3-quart baking dish, and add 1 cup frozen, defrosted and Dr.ained carrots, 1 cup.
- Cover and bake for 25 minutes.

- In a blending, bowl integrates1 cup biscuit mix and remaining 1/2 cup of skim milk. Stir till a soft dough types.
- Get rid of baking meal from oven and reveal.
- Spoon dough onto chicken and veggies with a tablespoon and spread evenly to cover the whole surface area of chicken mixture.
- Bake uncovered for 10 minutes, or until the biscuits are golden brown.

Broiled Chicken Kabobs

Active ingredients

- 1 tablespoon olive oil
- 1 teaspoon oregano
- 1 teaspoon basil
- 1/2 teaspoon rosemary
- 1/2 teaspoon parsley
- 1 1/2 pounds boneless, skinless chicken breast, cut into 1-inch pieces
- Nonstick veggie cooking spray
- 4 cups zucchini cut into 1-inch pieces
- 3 cups little whole button mushrooms, stems eliminated

- 1 cup long-grain wild rice, prepared according to directions without salt or fat

Preparation

- In a medium bowl, integrate 1 tablespoon olive oil, 1 teaspoon oregano, 1 teaspoon basil, 1/2 teaspoon rosemary and 1/2 teaspoon parsley.
- Add 1.5 pounds chicken pieces to a bowl and mix well, finish all sides of chicken.
- Let sit for 5 minutes.
- Spray a broiler pan with nonstick veggie spray.
- Stir 4 cups zucchini pieces and 3 cups button mushrooms into the bowl of the chicken mixture until well covered.
- Thread chicken, mushrooms, and zucchini pieces alternating them, on all 8 skewers.
- Place kabobs on broiler pan
- Broil 5 minutes on each side, turning when.
- Serve with hot wild rice.

Note: Kabobs are traditionally served over a bed of rice, with pita bread. They can be served on or off the skewer with dipping sauces of option.

Lighter Avocado Chicken Salad

Ingredients

- 1 big chicken breast (about 2 cups shredded)
- garlic powder, to taste
- newly cracked black pepper
- 1 small avocado, mashed
- 2 tablespoon plain nonfat Greek yoghurt
- 2 tablespoon lemon or lime juice
- 1/4 teaspoon garlic powder
- newly cracked pepper
- 1/2 cup diced onion, any kind
- 1/2 cup diced celery (about 1 rib)

Preparation

- Season chicken breast with garlic powder and pepper. Remove chicken and let cool before shredding.
- In a large bowl, smash avocado. Stir in yoghurt, lime juice, garlic powder and pepper. Stir in chicken, celery and onion. Shop in an airtight container in the fridge.

Tomato Basil Farro Salad

Ingredients

- 3 cups prepared farro, ready according to package directions
- 1 cup cherry tomatoes, cut in half
- 1/2 cup fresh basil leaves, sliced up thinly

- 1/3 cup fresh mozzarella (in small balls, halved, or one big one, cubed)
- 1 tablespoon olive oil
- 1 tablespoon balsamic vinegar
- 1 clove garlic, minced
- pinch freshly broken black pepper

Preparation

- In a big bowl, integrate farro, tomatoes, basil, and mozzarella.
- In a small bowl, blend together staying ingredients. Put over farro and carefully toss to coat. Serve immediately or refrigerate and cover approximately 2 days.

Lemon and Dill Zested Zucchini Salad

Active ingredients

- 2 medium zucchini, cut into ribbons with a vegetable peeler
- 1 cup of green peas
- 1 cup black beans
- 2 tablespoon dill, chopped
- zest from 1/2 lemon
- 1/2 teaspoon salt

Preparation

- Combine all of the ingredients in a small bowl. Chill before serving.

Cumin-Spiced Shredded Chicken, Barley, and Vegetable Soup

Ingredients

- 2 medium boneless, skinless chicken breast
- 1 tablespoon cumin
- 1 teaspoon Dr.ied oregano
- 1/2 teaspoon salt
- 1/2 cup barley
- 2 medium carrots, peeled and sliced
- 1 14-ounce can cannellini or other white beans washed
- 1 medium zucchini, spiralized
- 1 cup kale, sliced

Preparation

- Bring 8 cups of water to a boil and add the chicken breast, cumin, oregano, and salt. Boil, covered, until the chicken breast can easily be pierced through with a fork-- about 15 minutes.

- When ready, remove the chicken, pressure the liquid, and reserve for use as the base for the soup.
- Include barley to the strained liquid. Give a boil and cook, covered, for about 20 minutes.
- Add the carrots and beans and cook for another 10 to 15 minutes, up until the carrots are a little tender.
- On the other hand, shred the chicken. You can pull it apart using your hands or two forks.
- Stir in the chicken, zucchini, and kale. Simmer for another 5 minutes and serve.

Healthy Quinoa Stuffed Chicken Roll-Ups

Ingredients

- 2 tablespoons quinoa, Dr.y
- 1/2 medium carrot, julienned
- 1/4 cup broccoli stalks, julienned
- 2 medium boneless, skinless chicken breasts, pounded to 1/4" thickness
- 1/4 teaspoon salt
- 1/4 teaspoon oregano, Dr.y
- 1/2 cup spinach, sliced
- 2 tablespoons feta cheese, fallen apart
- Zest from 1/2 lemon

Preparation

- Set the quinoa to prepare according to package guidelines.
- Steam the carrots and broccoli stalks until a little tender.
- Preheat oven to 350F.
- Lay chicken breast flat on a lined baking sheet and gently spray with olive oil (or nonstick cooking spray) and rub with salt, on both sides.
- Divide the vegetables, oregano, and quinoa between the chicken breasts, in addition to the spinach, lemon enthusiasm, and feta cheese. Spoon whatever onto the middle, keeping the filling away from the edges, then start to roll from one end of the breast until you end up with a full roll. Tie with twine or insert toothpicks on either end to keep closed.
- Transfer the chicken rolls to a small heated pan, cooking up until golden brown on all sides, about 5 minutes.
- Transfer the rolls back to the baking sheet and continue cooking in the oven till the breasts are prepared through about 15 minutes.
- Let the chicken cool 5 minutes prior to slicing and serving.

Lean and Juicy Turkey and Mushroom Burgers

Ingredients

- 3/4 pound turkey breast, ground
- 1/2 cup child Bella mushrooms, carefully chopped
- 1 tablespoon olive oil
- 1 tablespoon Worcestershire sauce

Preparation

- Integrate the ground turkey breast, mushrooms, olive oil, and Worcestershire sauce in a small bowl.
- Divide the mixture into 6 parts and form a patty from each, about 1/2-inch thick, with your hands and set aside.
- Grease a stovetop frying pan or medium frying pan and cook the patties over medium heat, about 5 minutes on each side.

10-Minute Lemon-Zested Shrimp on Avocado Toast

Ingredients

- 8 medium shrimp (or 10 small shrimp), peeled and deveined
- 1/2 teaspoon olive oil
- 1/2 teaspoon lemon enthusiasm

- 1/8 teaspoon cumin
- 1 teaspoon cilantro, carefully sliced (optional)
- 2 pieces whole wheat bread
- 1/2 medium avocado, mashed
- pinch of salt (less than 1/8 teaspoon)
- 1/4 mango, thinly sliced

Preparation

- In a small bowl, integrate the shrimp with the olive oil, lemon passion, cumin, and optional cilantro.
- Heat a small frying pan over medium heat and add the shrimp. Cook for 4 to 5 minutes, flipping halfway.
- While the shrimp is cooking, toast the entire wheat bread slices and mash the avocado together with the salt.
- Spread out the avocado mash over the toasted bread and top with mango pieces, then shrimp.

Cod Parchment Packs

Active ingredients

- 2 cups sweet potato, julienned
- 1 pound cod, divided into 4 pieces
- 1 teaspoon Dr.ied thyme leaves

- 4 teaspoons olive oil
- 1 teaspoon kosher salt
- 4 slices of fresh lemon

Preparation

- Preheat oven to 400F.
- Fold 4 sheets of parchment paper in half.
- Include 1/4 of the sweet potatoes on one side of the parchment and top with a piece of cod.
- Spray each piece of fish with 1/4 teaspoon thyme, 1 teaspoon olive oil, 1/4 teaspoon, salt and a piece of lemon.
- Fold the parchment paper over the fish and vegetables, then fold and crease the edges to form a crescent and closed shaped package.
- Transfer packages to a flat pan and bake for 20 minutes.
- Eliminate from the oven and enable to rest for 5 minutes before tearing open.

Classic Pancakes With a Side of Red Delicious

Active ingredients

- 1/2 cup whole-wheat flour
- 1/2 cup all-purpose flour
- 1 tablespoon sugar

- 1 teaspoon baking powder
- 1/4 teaspoon salt
- 1 cup fat-free milk
- 1 large egg, beaten
- 2 tablespoons avocado, mashed
- 1 tablespoon water
- non-stick cooking spray
- 1 tablespoon saltless butter, melted
- 1 big red tasty apple
- 1/2 teaspoon ground ginger
- 1/2 teaspoon ground cinnamon
- 2 tablespoons water
- 1.5 teaspoons honey, divided

Preparation

- Integrate the Dr.y components (whole-wheat flour, all-purpose flour, sugar, baking powder, and salt) in a small bowl.
- Whisk together the wet ingredients (milk, egg, avocado, and water) in a different bowl, then contribute to the Dr.y components and stir up until well integrated.
- Spray a large pan with non-stick cooking spray and heat over a low-medium flame. Spoon the pancake batter into the pan, about 2 tablespoons per pancake, and flatten down into a round shape. Prepare for 2 to 3 minutes on one side

and an extra minute on the other, until slightly golden brown.

- While the pancakes are cooking, core and very finely slice the apple into 12 slices. In a bowl, pour the butter over the pieces and mix with the ginger and cinnamon.
- Organize the apple pieces in a separate pan and cook over medium flame for 3-5 minutes, until a little softened. Include the water midway through.
- Arrange 4 pancakes on a plate and top with the cooked apples. Sprinkle with 1/2 teaspoon honey and delight in.

Chicken Soup Noodle Bowl

Ingredients

- 2 cups low-sodium chicken broth
- 1-ounce Dr.y rice noodles
- 1/2 cup sugar snap peas
- 2 ounces of shredded chicken

Preparation

- Heat chicken broth in a small pan until simmering.
- Include rice noodles and cook, stirring periodically up until noodles hurt.
- Add snap peas and prepared chicken and simmer for an extra 2 to 3 minutes till snap peas are a little tender and all active ingredients are warmed through.
- Serve right away.

Broccoli and Cheese Stuffed Baked Potatoes

Ingredients

- 4 medium potatoes, baked, cut in half lengthwise
- 1 cup broccoli florets, chopped
- 1 cup low-fat cheddar cheese, shredded

Preparation

- Preheat oven to 350F.
- Place cut potatoes on a sheet pan, cut side up.
- Top each potato with broccoli and then spray with cheese.
- Bake for 10 to 15 minutes or up until cheese is melted.
- Enable to cool a little before serving.

Chicken Noodle Soup

Ingredients

- 1/2 tablespoon olive oil
- 1 cup sliced and cut celery
- 2 quarts water
- 2 cups peeled and sliced carrots
- 4 low-sodium chicken bouillon cubes
- 1/2 teaspoon thyme
- 1/2 teaspoon salt
- 3 ounces of raw egg noodles
- 2 cups diced, cooked boneless skinless chicken breasts
- 2 cups frozen peas

Preparation

- Add 1/2 tablespoon olive oil to a big pot. Include 2 cup cut and sliced celery and sauté over medium-high heat until translucent.
- Include 2 quarts water, 2 cups peeled and sliced carrots, 4 low-fat chicken bouillon cubes, 1/2 teaspoon thyme, and 1/2 teaspoon salt. Bring to a boil.
- Include 2 cups (3 ounces) large egg noodles to the boiling water. Stir. Go back to a boil, reduce

heat and cook for 8 minutes or until noodles are tender.

- Include 2 cups diced, cooked boneless skinless chicken breast meat and 2 cups frozen peas. Go back to a boil, reduce heat, cover and simmer over medium-low heat for 5 to 10 minutes.

Pantry Meals

Ingredients

- 2 slices whole-wheat or gluten-free bread
- 1 pound white fish (like halibut, cod or tilapia)
- 2 tsp Worcestershire sauce
- 2 tsp Dijon mustard
- 1 large egg
- 1rib celery (diced)
- 1/2 tsp grated lemon peel
- 2 Tbsp reduced-fat mayonnaise
- 1/2 tsp dried thyme
- 1/8 tsp salt
- fresh ground black pepper (to taste)
- 2 Tbsp extra virgin olive oil

Direction

- Toast bread until lightly browned. Let cool and procedure in mini chopper or blender.

- Coarsely chop the fish. This can be carried out in the food processor, but with care or the fish will rapidly turn into a paste.
- Fold the fish together with the breadcrumbs. Include Worcestershire sauce, mustard, egg, celery, lemon peel, mayo, thyme, pepper and salt.
- Fold together carefully up until well blended.
- Kind into 8 cakes and chill. This can be made up to 12 hours ahead of time.
- Preheat the oven to 325 ° F.
- Place the oil in a large non-stick frying pan over high heat up until the oil is almost cigarette smoking.
- Place cakes in the hot oil and cook over medium-high heat for about 3 minutes up until brown. Cook and turn for about 2 minutes. Place in a hot oven. Cook for another 9-- 10 minutes.

Fish Soup with Yams

Active ingredients

- 1 Tbsp olive oil
- 1 large onion (diced)

- 2ribs celery (diced)
- 1 large carrot (peeled and diced)
- 16 ounces yams (peeled and diced)
- 2anchovy filets (canned in water is finest) (minced)
- 5 cups of water
- 1/2lemon (juiced)
- 2bay leaves
- 1/2 tsp Dried marjoram
- 1/4 tsp salt
- fresh ground black pepper (to taste)
- 2 cloves garlic.
- 16 ounces firm white fish (like cod, Mahi or halibut Mahi)

Direction

- Place the olive oil in a medium stockpot over medium heat. Add the onion and cook for about 2 minutes, stirring frequently.
- Add the celery and carrots and cook for two minutes. Include the yams and cook for one minute.
- Include the anchovies, water, lemon juice, bay leaves, salt, marjoram and pepper.
- Add the 2 cloves to the pot. Stir occasionally and prepare for about 45 minutes.

- Cut the fish into 1-inch cubes and add to the soup. Cook for another 20 minutes. Remove the garlic cloves and bay leaves prior to serving.

Ginger Papaya Whitefish

Active ingredients

- 1 tsp sesame oil
- 1/2 tsp ground ginger
- 1/4 cup papaya juice
- 1/4 tsp salt
- fresh ground black pepper (to taste)
- spray olive oil
- 26-ounce whitefish filets (cod, orange roughy or tilapia)
- 1 tsp corn starch
- 4 Tbsp water
- 2 Tbsp fresh cilantro leaves

Direction

- Put the sesame oil, ground ginger, papaya juice, salt and pepper in a small mixing bowl and whisk till well mixed.
- Place a big non-stick skillet on the variety over medium-high heat. When the pan is hot spray lightly with olive oil. Include the fish filets.

Cook for about 4 minutes on one side and after that turn.

- After cooking the fish for about 3 minutes blend the cornstarch with the 4 tablespoons of water in a little dish up until well combined. Add the cornstarch mixture to the papaya sauce and blend well.
- Add the papaya sauce to the pan with the fish. When and get rid of the fish to serving plates, turn the fish. Blend the sauce well and divide uniformly over the fish filets.
- Sprinkle with cilantro leaves and serve.

Ginger Peanut Whitefish

Active ingredients

- 4 tsp sesame oil
- 1 clove garlic (minced)
- 1 large shallot (minced)
- 1/4 cup raw saltless peanuts (shelled)
- 3 Tbsp fresh ginger (minced)
- 1/2lime (juiced)
- 1/2 tsp sugar
- 1 Tbsp low salt soy or gluten-free tamari sauce
- fresh ground black pepper (to taste).
- 1 cup low sodium chicken broth
- 4-ounce white fish filets (halibut, grouper, cod)

Instructions

- Pour 3 teaspoons of the sesame oil in a little skillet over medium heat. Add the garlic and cook for about 3 minutes.
- Include the peanuts and shallots. Cook for another 3 minutes, stirring sometimes.
- Add the ginger and cook for another 3-- 5 minutes. Include the lime juice, sugar, soy chicken, sauce and pepper stock.
- Minimize the heat up until the sauce is simmering. Cook for about 10 minutes is decreasing by about 1/2.
- When the sauce is done, reduce the heat to low to keep warm.
- Place a large non-stick skillet over medium-high heat. When the pan is hot, include the fish.
- Serve the fish topped with sauce.

Halibut with Cilantro Ginger Sauce

Active ingredients

- 1 Tbsp sesame oil
- 1 medium shallot (minced)
- 2 Tbsp fresh ginger (minced)
- 1/2 cup low sodium chicken broth
- 1/4 tsp salt
- fresh ground black pepper
- 1/2 cup fresh cilantro leaves
- 1 tsp unsalted butter

- spray olive oil
- 4 4 ounce halibut fillets

Direction

- Place a big skillet in the oven and preheat to 425 ° F. Place the sesame oil in a little frying pan over medium heat. Include the shallot and cook for about 3 minutes till simply clear.
- Include the minced ginger and cook for another three minutes. Add the chicken stock, salt, pepper and stir. Simmer for about 15 minutes.
- Place the sauce in a blender and include the fresh cilantro. Add the butter and permit to melt.
- Spray the big frying pan with oil and add the halibut skin side down. Roast for about 10-- 14 minutes until done. Serve topped with the sauce.

Halibut with Dill and Potato Topping

Ingredients

- 2-quart water
- 12 ounces small red potatoes
- 2 4 ounce halibut fillets
- 2 Tbsp fresh dill
- 1/8 tsp Dried tarragon

- 1/4 tsp salt
- fresh ground black pepper
- 2 tsp unsalted butter
- spray olive oil
- 1/4 cup water
- 2 Tbsp fresh lemon juice

Instructions

- Pour the water in a big stockpot over high heat. Include the potatoes and cook until the water has actually been boiling for about 8 to 10 minutes.
- Get rid of the potatoes and rinse under cold water. Slice as very finely as you can.
- Place a large frying pan in the oven and preheat the oven to 425 ° F. Rinse the halibut filets under cold water and pat Dr.y. Place on a cutting board skin side down. Spread out the dill throughout the top of the fish and after that spray with the pepper, tarragon and salt.
- Gently layer the potatoes on the fish beginning at one end and overlapping till the fish is covered. Top each of the fish with 1/2 teaspoon of the butter (save the other teaspoon for later).
- Spray the frying pan gently with olive oil and place the fish in the pan skin side down. Prepare for about 6 minutes and after that spray the fish

lightly with olive oil and alter the setting of the oven to broil. Prepare for about 4 more minutes and remove the pan from the oven.
- Place the fish on plates and put the hot pan on the variety over medium heat. Blend in, and put the sauce over the fish and serve.

Halibut with Peanut Cilantro Butter

Ingredients

- 3 Tbsp unsalted butter
- 1 Tbsp peanut butter
- 2 Tbsp fresh cilantro
- 1/4 tsp rice vinegar
- 1 Tbsp low-sodium soy sauce
- 24-ounce halibut filets
- fresh ground black pepper

Instructions

- Mix the spread together with the peanut butter, vinegar, cilantro and soy sauce. This can be done up to 24 hours ahead of time and kept in the refrigerator.
- Preheat oven to 425 ° F. Place a big skillet in the oven.

- Season the halibut with the pepper if you want and position the filets in the pan. Return the pan to the oven and cook for about 5 minutes and then turn.

Halibut with Rosemary Maple Glaze

Ingredients

- 2 small white onions
- 2 tsp fresh rosemary leaves
- 1/2 cup low sodium chicken or veggie broth
- 1/4 tsp salt
- 2 Tbsp maple syrup
- 2 Tbsp unsalted butter
- fresh ground black pepper
- 24-ounce halibut filets (without skin)
- spray olive or grapeseed oil

Directions

- Preheat the oven to 325 ° F. Place the peeled white onions in a medium saucepan, cover and location the pan in the oven.

- While the onions are cooking combine the rosemary leaves, chicken maple, stock and salt syrup in a little saucepan.
- Place the pan over medium heat and prepare the sauce up until it is lowered by half. This will take about 15 minutes.
- After another 20 minutes, position a medium-sized frying pan in the oven and increase the heat to 400 ° F. Season the fish with the pepper. Lightly spray the frying pan with oil and location the halibut in the pan. Return the pan to the oven and cook for about 4 minutes.
- Remove the fish and turn them over. Include the reduced rosemary maple glaze to the pan and return the pan to the oven. Prepare for another 5 - 6 minutes.
- Put an onion in the centre of a plate and top it with the cooked halibut filet. Pour the glaze over the top and serve.

Maple Glazed Salmon with Lentils

Ingredients

- spray olive oil
- 1 large rib celery (diced)
- 2 medium carrots (peeled and diced)
- 1/2 cup red lentils
- 1 cup of water

- 1/2 cup low salt chicken or veggie broth
- 1/4 tsp salt
- 1 tsp Dried marjoram
- fresh ground black pepper (to taste)
- 1 Tbsp extra virgin olive oil
- 24-ounce salmon filets
- 2 Tbsp maple syrup

Instructions

- Place a medium frying pan over medium heat and spray lightly with olive oil. Include the celery and carrots and cook, stirring often, for about 5 minutes.
- Include the water, chicken stock, salt and marjoram. Prepare for about 20 - 25 minutes up until the lentils are simply soft.
- When the lentils have to do with midway done preheat the oven to 375 ° F. Place a frying pan in the oven.
- When the lentils are done, add the olive oil, stir and decrease the heat to low.
- Leading with one tablespoon of maple syrup and return the pan to the oven for about 4 minutes. Cook for another 4 - 6 minutes.
- Serve the lentils topped with the cooked salmon. There will be a little sauce in the bottom of the skillet, and this goes over the salmon.

Molasses Glazed Salmon

Ingredients

- 1 Tbsp molasses or black treacle
- 1/8 tsp cayenne pepper
- 1/8 tsp salt
- 1/2 tsp white wine vinegar
- 1/2 tsp smoked paprika
- 1 Tbsp olive oil
- 2 4 ounce salmon fillets (skinless)

Direction

- Whisk together the molasses, cayenne pepper, salt, vinegar and paprika.
- Place a big frying pan in the oven and preheat to 400 ° F
- . When the pan is hot, add the olive oil to the pan and then the salmon filets.
- Spoon the molasses glaze over the fish and roast for about 13 to 15 minutes.
- Serve.

Mustard Seared Whitefish

Ingredients

- 1 large egg

- 3 tsp olive oil
- 2 tsp dijon mustard
- 1/8 tsp salt
- 1/8 tsp paprika
- 1 TbspDr.ied sage
- fresh ground black pepper
- 2 4 ounce white fish filets (trout, cod, Dr.um, or tilapia)

Direction

- Blend together the egg, 1 teaspoon of the olive oil, Dijon mustard, salt, paprika, sage and black pepper till smooth. Put the mix in the refrigerator.
- Place a large frying pan in the oven and preheat to 400 ° F
- While the oven is preheating rinse the fish filets and pat Dr.y with a paper towel.
- When the oven is hot, include the remaining 2 teaspoons of olive oil to the pan. Dr.edge both sides of the fish in the mustard finish and place them in the hot pan.
- Return the pan to the oven and cook for about 4 minutes on the first side. Modification the setting of the oven to broil and cook for about another 3 - 4 minutes.

Oven-Fried Fish

Ingredients

- 1 large egg
- 1 large egg white
- 1 TbspDijon mustard.
- 1box (5 ounces) plain melba toast
- 1/4 tsp salt
- 1/2 tsp ground black pepper
- 44-ounce fish filets (tilapia, cod, whiting)
- Spray oil

Instructions

- Preheat oven to 375 ° F. Place a big non-stick cookie sheet or skillet in the oven.
- Place the fish filets on a stack of three paper towels so that they are not touching each other. Cover with there more paper towels and push down somewhat so that as much of the fish touches with the towel.
- Place the egg, egg white and Dijon mustard in a small bowl. Blend up until smooth.
- In a food mill fitted with a steel blade, position the melba toast, salt and black pepper and

process until small crumbs. Leave some pieces about the size of currants.

- Dr.edge a fish filet in the egg mixture, coating completely. Dr.edge in the breadcrumbs, patting and turning regularly till well layered.
- Dig up the layered fish in the egg clean a 2nd time and then coat again with breadcrumbs.
- Place the fish in the pan so that the fillets do not touch each other. Spray the top of the fish gently and then place in oven. Spray the top of each fish filet lightly with the oil.

Pecan Crusted Trout

Ingredients

- 1 1/2 ounces raw pecans
- 1 Tbsp fresh sage
- 1 1/2 tsp fresh rosemary
- 1/8 tsp salt
- fresh ground black pepper (to taste)
- 1/4 tsp smoked paprika
- 1 Tbsp maple syrup
- 2 4 ounce boneless trout filets (skin on)
- 1 Tbsp olive oil
- 1/4 cup white wine
- 1 tsp unsalted butter

Instructions

- Place the pecans, sage, rosemary, salt, pepper, and paprika in a mini-chopper or mixer and pulse until the mixture is the consistency of coarse sand. (The pecans need to be about the size of Dried quinoa - smaller sized than Dr.ied lentils.).
- Place the pecan mixture in a little bowl and include the maple syrup. Fold together up until well combined.
- Place a big skillet in the oven and preheat the oven to 375F.
- Place the trout skin side down on a small plate or cutting board. Pat the pecan mixture evenly onto the flesh side of the trout.
- When the oven is hot, include the olive oil to the pan and return to the oven (to heat up the oil). After 1 minute, position the trout fillets in the pan, skin side down, and return the pan to the oven. Cook the fish for 5 minutes.
- Set the oven to broil.
- Broil the fish for 3-5 minutes, or until the crust is lightly browned.
- Remove the pan from the oven and place the trout filets on different dinner plates.
- Place the pan on the stove over medium-high heat.
- Include the Gewurztraminer to the pan, swirl for 30-45 seconds, and add the butter. Stir until

melted, and leading the trout fillets with the sauce.

- Serve.

Roasted Trout with Sage Pecan Granola

Ingredients

- 1 1/2 ounces raw pecans
- 1 tsp.rubbed, Dr.ied sage
- 1/4 tsp Dried rosemary
- 1/8 tsp salt
- to taste fresh ground black pepper
- 1/4 tsp smoked paprika
- 1/4 cup panko breadcrumbs or gluten-free panko breadcrumbs
- 1 Tbsp.maple syrup
- 2 4-ounce boneless trout filets (skin on)
- 1 Tbsp.olive oil

Instructions

- Place a little skillet over medium-high heat.
- Include the pecans and toast them, toss regularly. Change the heat so the pecans brown, however, does not burn.
- Place the toasted pecans, sage, rosemary, salt, pepper, and paprika in a mini-chopper or

blender and pulse till the mixture is the consistency of 1/8 inch pebbles. (This should just be a couple of pulses.).

- Place the pecan mix in a small bowl and add the breadcrumbs. Fold together until well mixed.
- Place a big frying pan in the oven and preheat the oven to 375F.
- When the pan is hot, include 1 teaspoon of oil to the pan.
- Add the pecan-breadcrumb mix to the skillet and toast for about 10 minutes. Toss periodically and remove from the oven when the mix is golden brown.
- Remove to a bowl and set aside. Return the pan to the oven.
- Place the trout skin side down on a little plate or cutting board.
- Brush the top (the skinless side) with the maple syrup.
- Include the oil to the pan and after that the trout, skin side down.
- Prepare the fish for 5 minutes.
- Modification of the oven temperature to broil.
- Broil the fish for 3-5 minutes, or till the crust is lightly browned.
- Remove the pan from the oven and place the trout filets on separate dinner plates.
- Leading with the pecan granola and serve.

Pork Tenderloin with Barley Casserole

Active ingredients

- 4 Tbsp unsalted butter
- 1 medium onion (diced)
- 1 large carrot (peeled and diced)
- 1 lb crimini mushroom (sliced)
- 1/2 large red bell pepper (diced)
- 1 cup barley
- 1/2 tsp salt
- 1 Tbsp fresh sage (minced)
- fresh ground black pepper (to taste)
- 1 lb pork tenderloin (cut into 1/2 inch cubes).
- 2 cups low sodium chicken or vegetable broth
- 1/2 cup water

Instructions

- Preheat the oven to 325 ° F. Place the light spread in a big saucepan or medium Dutch oven over medium heat.
- When the spread is melted, add the onion and carrot. Prepare for about 5 minutes, stirring frequently, till the onion is somewhat soft.
- Include the mushrooms and cook, tossing often, till the mushrooms are gently browned.

- Add the red bell pepper, barley, salt, pepper, pork and sage. Stir and add the chicken stock and water.
- Stir and cover the pot and after that place in the oven. Inspect about every 14 minutes to make certain that there suffices liquid. Include water 1/4 cup at a time as required. Overall cooking time will be about 45 - 60 minutes, or up until the barley hurts but not gummy.

Asian Peanut Chicken with Noodles

Ingredients

- 3 quartswater
- 3 Tbsp smooth peanut butter
- 1/4 cup fresh cilantro leaves
- 1/2lime (juiced)
- 2 tsp low-sodium soy sauce
- 2 Tbsp low sodium chicken or veggie broth
- 1/8 tsp red pepper flakes
- 6 ounces boneless skinless chicken breast (sliced into strips)
- 1/2 cup frozen edamame (soybeans)
- 4 ounces whole wheat or gluten-free spaghetti
- 1 small carrot (shredded)
- red onion (slivered; to taste)
- 2 Tbsp Dried roasted unsalted peanuts

Direction

- Place peanut butter, cilantro, lime juice, soy sauce, chicken stock, and red pepper flakes in a mixer or mini chopper and puree up until smooth. Reserve.
- Preheat oven to 200 °
- Place 3 quarts water in a large pan over high heat. When water boils, decrease the heat to medium until water is simmering. Add chicken strips and cook for 5 minutes. Get rid of the chicken with tongs, leaving the water in the pot, and put the plate in the preheated oven.
- Increase the heat under the water to high, and when the water goes back to a boil, add the whole wheat pasta. Cook for 8-10 minutes, until pasta is nearly al dente. Add edamame and cook for another 1 minute.
- Decrease the heat to medium and add peanut sauce, chicken, and shredded onions and carrots, then toss well. (Don't include onions if they are a GERD trigger for you).
- If the sauce is too thick, add the reserved pasta water, one tablespoon at a time, up until it reaches the wanted consistency. Leading with peanuts and serve.

Chicken Saltimbocca

Ingredients

- 2 4 ounce chicken breasts
- 4 1/2 ounce pieces prosciutto
- 8 large leaves fresh sage (chiffonade)
- fresh ground black pepper
- 1 Tbsp olive oil
- 8 ounces crimini mushrooms (quartered)
- 1 large shallot (minced)
- 1/4 cup low salt chicken or veggie broth
- 1 tsp unsalted butter
- 3 quartswater
- 4 ounces whole wheat or gluten-free angel hair pasta

Instructions

- Place the chicken breasts flat on a cutting board and slice them into two thinner pieces. Place the chicken breast slices between sheets of plastic wrap. Utilizing a flat meat mallet, pound them carefully till they are about 1/8 to 1/4 inch thick.
- Spray each chicken breast with pepper and then place a piece of prosciutto ham on each flattened breast. Uniformly spread out the sage in between the 4 chicken breasts, putting it on top of the prosciutto. Roll the chicken breast up around the ham and sage.
- Set the covered chicken bundles aside in the fridge till ready to utilize.

- Preheat the oven to 325 ° F. Place a large non-stick frying pan over medium-high heat. Add the olive oil, shallots and mushrooms and cook, stirring regularly, until browned. Add the rolled chicken breasts to the pan and sear on each side, then remove them to a pan or piece of foil and place them in the oven.
- Add the chicken stock to the skillet and minimize the heat to medium. Include the butter and decrease the heat to low.
- Pour the water in a large saucepan over high heat. Add the pasta when it begins to boil.
- When the pasta is done, remove the angel hair using tongs and place it in the frying pan with the mushroom sauce. Add 1/4 cup of the pasta water and increase the heat to medium-high. Toss the pasta well for about a minute.
- Serve the pasta with the sauce and location the chicken on top.

Chicken Satay

Active ingredients

- 4skewers
- 1 tsp sugar
- 1/4 tsp salt
- 1 Tbsp curry powder
- 1/2 cup light coconut milk

- fresh ground black pepper (to taste)
- 1 lb boneless skinless chicken breast (cut into 4 4-ounce strips)
- spray oil

Instructions

- If utilizing wood skewers, put them in a big meal with water to soak so that they don't burn while cooking.
- Place the sugar, salt, curry powder, coconut milk and pepper in a small bowl and blend till smooth.
- Thread the chicken slices onto the skewers. Put the chicken in the bottom of a big enough dish to enable them to all lay flat (I used a rectangular Pyrex dish). Leading with the satay marinade. Marinate for a minimum of 30 minutes (overnight is best, but a half-hour approximately will do).
- Place a non-stick frying pan on the range over medium-high heat. Spray gently with oil and place the skewered chicken on the frying pan.
- Cook on each side about 8-- 10 minutes, till prepared through. After each turn of the chicken baste with a little of the staying marinade.
- Serve the chicken over Coconut Rice and top with Thai Peanut Sauce.

Chinese Chicken Salad

Active ingredients

- 3 quartswater
- 8 ounces whole wheat or gluten-free udon noodles
- 2 tsp dark sesame oil
- 4 ounces shiitake mushrooms (thinly sliced)
- spray oil
- 1/4 cup slivered almonds
- 16 ounces boneless skinless chicken breast
- 1 Tbsp low-sodium soy sauce
- 8 ounces napa cabbage (thinly sliced)
- 8 ounces carrots (peeled and very finely sliced)
- 4 ounces snow peas
- 3 Tbsp hoisin sauce
- 2 Tbsp rice vinegar
- 2 Tbsp pineapple juice
- 111-ounce can mandarin oranges (Dr.ained pipes)
- 2 tsp black sesame seeds (optional)

Direction

- Place the water in a medium stockpot over high heat.

- When water boils, add the udon noodles and cook for 6-8 minutes. Dr.ain pipes, getting rid of excess water, then place in a large blending bowl. Include sesame oil, toss until layered, then Place in the refrigerator.
- Place a large frying pan over medium-high heat while the water is about boiling. Sprinkle softly with oil and mushrooms in slices. Cook the champagne until brown. Toss frequently. Continue cooking with and include almonds until they are gently browned. Release the heat and reserve.
- Cook the oven up to 375 and put in an oven with a large saucepan. Sprinkle the pot lightly with oil when preheated and add the chicken breasts. Prepare and turn the chicken for 8 minutes. Serve the soy and cook for 5-7 minutes or until the chicken has been cooked.
- Once cooked, get rid of chicken from the oven and cut into 1/4 inch strips. Chill.
- While you are cooking chicken, in a small bowl chill with hoisin sauce, rice vinegar, and pineapple juice.
- Fold together with udon nodes, sweet chops, carrots, snow peas and Dr.essing when the chicken is cool. The mushroom and almond blend and the mandarin oranges are on top of the line. Attach sesame seeds to the garnish.

Mango Chicken Salad

Active ingredients

- 4 cups of water
- 1 lb boneless skinless chicken breasts
- 2 large ribs celery (diced)
- 1 large mango (peeled and diced)
- 1/2red bell pepper (diced)
- 1/4 cup slivered almonds
- 2 Tbsp fresh dill
- 1/2 cup reduced-fat mayo
- 2 Tbsp orange juice.
- 1/4 tsp salt
- fresh ground black pepper (to taste)

Instructions

- Pour the water in a large skillet over medium heat. Bring the water to a boil and after that reduce the heat till the water is at a shiver.
- Carefully add the chicken breasts and poach for about 10 - 15 minutes depending on the thickness of the breasts. It's finest to utilize an instantaneous thermometer and remove the breasts just as they reach 160 ° F.
- Let the chicken rest for about 5 - 10 minutes. When they are cool, cut them into 1/2 inch

cubes. Chill in the refrigerator for about 30 minutes.

- Get rid of the chicken from the fridge and add the diced celery, mango, red bell pepper, almonds, mayo, dill, orange juice, salt and pepper. Fold the salad together carefully and chill for another 15 minutes (or overnight).
- Serve.

Mushroom Salad

Active ingredients

- 1 Tbsp olive oil
- 2 tsp coarse ground mustard
- 2 tsp white wine vinegar
- 2 Tbsp reduced-fat sour cream
- 2 Tbsp2% milk
- 1/8 tsp salt
- fresh ground black pepper (to taste)
- 1/2 tsp fresh orange passion
- 8 ounces white mushrooms (sliced)
- 2leaves Romaine lettuce

Direction

- Whisk the olive oil together with the mustard, vinegar, sour cream, pepper, salt and milk. Include orange enthusiasm, Chill.
- Slice the mushrooms very thin when ready to be served. Toss the Dr.essing together.
- Up the roman flag, serve.

NATURAL CURES FOR ACID REFLUX: HEALTHY ACID REFLUX TREATMENT

Some of the most effective all-natural treatments for indigestion entail easy points like consuming raw foods, while other treatments are more intricate.

Below are a couple of natural cures to help you do away with your acid reflux without needing medication.

- **Eat Raw Foods**

Raw foods have a specific enzyme which your body needs in order to control food digestion and food distribution. However, these enzymes are reduced to a low of 116 degrees, Fahrenheit the temperature of your food.

If you want to undergo an extra-efficient reflux treatment of acid, try getting even more raw foods (not the food mentioned above) to increase your body's enzymes.

- **Get More Vitamin D**

Vitamin D is a vital vitamin for lots of functions in your body, and it assists in creating special peptides in your tummy that will aid to treat infections in your body (such as in the oesophagus).

You can obtain great deals of Vitamin D from the sunlight (watch out for radiation), yet you can also find lots of excellent foods and also supplements that are rich in the necessary vitamin.

- **Exercise More**

That's right: exercise is vital to virtually every little thing, and also it might make fairly a distinction if you include it in your heartburn treatment.

If you wish to improve your body's natural defences against heartburn and GERD, get out of your house and do at least 30 minutes of moderate exercise 5 times a week.

It will certainly assist you to lose weight, improve your blood circulation, enhance your body's gastrointestinal system, control your metabolic process, as well as eradicate your heartburn.

Heartburn Treatment(Herbal Acid Reflux Remedies)

There are some pretty incredible natural heartburn treatments that you may wish to take into consideration if your stomach acid is breaking down.

However, each GERD condition is different, and what may benefit some, may not help others. Simply put, when it pertains to food, a little bit of experimentation is probably inevitable.

- **Apple Cider Vinegar**

Apple cider vinegar contains pectin, which is among the best fat loss substances. The vinegar will also help to calm your inadequate roiling tummy, and also will certainly assist in protecting against the extremely severe pain that is caused by acid reflux. It is a fast-acting treatment that can decrease as well as stop the pain.

- **Baking Soda**

So, many people have heard about the numerous benefits of sodium bicarbonate, and one of the benefits is to help treat heart and indigestion. In fact, it is among the components of antacids and can help to stop stomach discomfort simply by adding a dose of it to a glass of water.

- **Fennel Seeds**

Fennel seeds are superb for aiding to handle GERD as well as heartburn, as it aids to reduce the acid in your belly. As long as you aren't expectant, it is an exceptional treatment to think about.

- **Peppermint**

Did you know that peppermint can assist in resolving your tummy and also calming the acid that is churning inside your gastrointestinal system? This is why many physicians suggest a peppermint after consuming. However, you ought to recognize that it may cause an increase in acid manufacturing before it helps your tummy to settle down.

- **German Chamomile**

This is a yummy herb that has actually been given for centuries as a therapy to help work out sleep-deprived children down. However, it can additionally assist in soothing your bad digestive system down and reduce the swelling of your digestive tract.

- **Meadowsweet**

Meadowsweet, when prepared in the form of a tea, can provide relief from the discomfort of heartburn. It is a natural herb that can soothe and also cool your inadequate tummy and oesophagus, and also will certainly help to cut down on the production of acid while decreasing swelling.

These are a few easy natural herbal solutions that might work for your all-natural heartburn treatment, and also they are worth thinking about if you are really feeling the discomfort that accompanies GERD and also heartburn.

You may not have a long-term outcome. They can certainly help, however, to reduce the pain that you really feel.

ACID REFLUX BENEFITS

When the sphincter muscle at the base of your oesophagus gets weak as well as stays too unwinded when it should not, GERD takes place. That enables acid from your belly to support right into your oesophagus, creating continuous signs such as heartburn, cough, and ingesting problems. In even more difficult situations, GERD can cause vomiting, respiratory system issues, constricting of your oesophagus, and also boosted the danger of oesophagus cancer cells.

The GERD diet plan helps your lower oesophagus sphincter muscle mass job better and also stay closed after you eat, so you'll have less of these concerns.

To achieve this, the GERD diet plan focuses on staying clear of foods that research has actually shown are most likely to trigger reflux as well as your signs. These are mostly foods that are acidic and/or high in fat.2 (Note, nevertheless, that staying clear of trigger foods totally still will not guarantee GERD administration).

In addition to increasing stomach acid, high-fat dishes postpone stomach Dr.aining and cause the muscles in the lower oesophagus to kick back, resulting in heartburn. Foods that are really acidic can be specifically bothersome to your stomach and also the oesophagus.

Boosting fibre is likewise advised. In a study published worldwide Journal of Gastroenterology, higher-fibre diet regimens increased oesophagus sphincter stress, lowered the number times acid supported, and lowered the variety of heartburn cases. To check the concept, researchers asked people with heartburn to add 15 grams of a psyllium fibre supplement daily-- as well as it functioned.

A 2016 research study published in Diseases of the Oesophagus discovered that consuming a Mediterranean-style diet is associated with a reduced threat of GERD.

That makes good sense because the Mediterranean diet plan is known for being reduced in fatty meats and also refined foods, and also greater in seafood, fruits, veggies, seeds, beans, and also nuts.

In addition to enhancing your signs, in this manner of consuming might cause some weight loss. Being overweight puts you at a much greater risk of GERD, as well as much research study has found that reducing weight is just one of the most effective methods to avoid the problem. Just a 10% reduction in weight boosts GERD symptoms and commonly permits people to go off prescribed acid blocker Dr.ugs (with their doctor's authorization).

Which Types of Doctors Treat Acid Reflux? When Should You See One

Several individuals can ease their reflux condition signs by adjustments in their routines, diet plan, and lifestyle, others need to consult their health-care specialist.

A gastroenterologist, an expert in stomach (GI) disorders, can be referred to. You will certainly be a simple doctor if your signs and symptoms are severe, and also if you are having surgery.

Call your health-care professional when symptoms of GERD happen frequently, disrupt your rest, interfere with work or other tasks, are connected with respiratory troubles, or are not eliminated by self-care procedures alone.

Make your health-care expert conscious that you are using self-care procedures or over the counter medicines so that they can keep an eye on exactly how well they work as well as exactly how frequently you require to utilize them.

If you have any of the following, go right away to the emergency situation division where you will certainly be seen by an emergency situation medical professional:

- Extreme chest pain or stress, especially if it emits to your arm, neck, or back
- Throwing up followed by serious breast pain
- Throwing up blood
- Dark, tarry stools
- Trouble swallowing
- Lack of breath

HOME REMEDIES TREAT AND SOOTH ACID REFLUX

For some individuals, indigestion signs might be soothed by transforming habits, diet regimen, as well as lifestyle. The following actions might lower reflux.

There are some quite amazing natural remedy for acid reflex therapy, as well as these treatments will certainly be wonderful to try if you are really feeling the pain from acid reflux, GERD or heart shed:

- Do not consume within 3 hours of going to bed. This permits your tummy to empty and acid manufacturing to lower.
- Do not lie down right after eating at any time of day.
- Elevate the head of your bed 6 inches with blocks. Gravity helps avoid reflux.
- Don't eat large meals. Consuming a lot of food at once enhances the quantity of acid required to absorb it. Consume smaller, much more constant meals throughout the day.
- Stay clear of fatty or oily foods, delicious chocolate, caffeine, mints or mint-flavoured foods, spicy foods, citrus, and tomato-based foods. These foods lower the proficiency of the reduced oesophagus sphincter (LES).
- Avoid alcohol consumption alcohol. Alcohol increases the possibility that acid from your stomach will certainly support.

- Quit cigarette smoking. Smoking cigarettes weakens the lower oesophagus sphincter and also increases reflux.
- Shed excess weight. Overweight and also overweight people are far more most likely to have annoying reflux than people of healthy weight.
- Stand upright or stay up straight, preserve great pose. This aids food and acid go through the stomach instead of backing up right into the oesophagus.
- Speak to your medical specialist about taking pain relievers like aspirin, Advil (Advil, Motrin), or osteoporosis medication on an over-the-counter basis. In some cases, these can exacerbate reflux.
- Talk with your health-care professional if you require pointers on reducing weight or giving up cigarette smoking.

Aloe Vera

Aloe Vera is understood for its soothing as well as relaxing effect, as well as it will aid to calm the pain in your oesophagus as well as stomach.

It also aids to boost your food digestion, so mix up some aloe vera juice in water to provide your stomach with a break.

Liquorice

Liquorice can be really reliable at helping to shield your tummy from acid reflux, as it produces a thick gel that lines the inside of your tummy.

This isn't the Twizzlers that you discover in Walmart, but it is the herbal liquorice that has been made use of as a herbal solution for centuries.

Papaya

As mentioned above, papaya can be effective in lowering the pain from indigestion. However, you may not have fresh papaya fruit if you do not stay in the tropics.

You can normally locate chewable tablets in the pharmacy, and they will certainly be effective at helping to treat your heartburn.

Periodontal

Chewing gum tissue will really assist to decrease the pain of acid reflux, as the enhanced saliva production triggered by your eating will aid to relieve your bad oesophagus, trigger the acid to be reduced the effects of, and also send the acid back down into your tummy thanks to the fact that you are frequently swallowing.

HEARTBURN MEDICATION

Here are several of the medicines you might wish to consider if acid reflux is a major issue:

- **Antacids**

Antacids are the short term option to heartburn, as they aid to send out the acid on down into your intestinal tracts. The effects last for an hour or two before the acid begins building up.

Foam Barriers

Foam barriers work like antacids, yet they also produce a foamy surface area in addition to the acid that stops it from coming back up. It is a much more long term remedy.

H2 Antagonists

These H2 blockers primarily avoid the belly from producing acid, hence providing a much more long term remedy.

PPI

Proton pump inhibitors shut off the secretion of acid in your belly for an extended period of time, thus offering a lot more long-term remedy to heartburn.

Pro-Motility Dr.ugs

These Dr.ugs reinforce the muscles of your gastrointestinal system to aid relocate the food as well as acid along with its method.

Medicines are often the way to opt for your indigestion therapy, though not constantly.

ONE-OF-A-KIND ACID REFLUX CURES (THE ACID REFLUX PILLOW)

The heartburn cushion is a cool invention, as well as it can be really efficient in assisting in preventing indigestion from embedding in during the night.

The cushion generally appears like a comfortable ramp, and also it raises your head a minimum of 45 levels over your tummy. This aids to avoid belly acid from returning up, as gravity works to maintain the acid heading in the direction of your intestinal tracts rather than back up your oesophagus.

Moderation is the Key to the GERD Diet for GERD Treatment

The trick to the GERD diet plan is, in fact, to reduce the food you consume, as that is the most reliable heartburn treatment.

The less food in your belly, the less acidity your tummy needs to produce and the less pressure on your oesophagus.

CONCLUSION

While there are a myriad of medicines on the market now to treat reflux expenditures in the United States for Dr.ugs such as proton pump inhibitors (PPIs) amount to $7 billion a year-- many people either do not wish to depend on medicines or are worried about possible adverse effects.

It's crucial to care for reflux, also called GERD or gastro oesophagus reflux condition. Symptoms consist of heartburn, regurgitation, sour taste in the mouth, and/or breast pain. The pain and also discomfort from GERD can adversely impact many aspects of your life, including your sleep and efficiency at the workplace. Chronic GERD is likewise a threat element for the growth of major problems such as Barrett's oesophagus (a precancerous modification of the cellular lining of the oesophagus) as well as also oesophagus cancer. You might be amazed to discover what you do as well as don't need to do to treat it.

DISCLAIMER

This book is not meant to replace doctors ' medical advice. The reader will consult a doctor periodically for health issues and, in particular, for any signs that may need treatment or medical attention.

(Health, nutrition)

Don't go, one final thing to do!!!

I would be extremely thankful if you had a quick review of Amazon if you liked this book or found it useful. Your support makes a difference and I personally read all the reviews so I can get your feedback and improve this book.

Thanks for your support again! Thanks!